Advance praise

'*Trying to Conceive* is a delightful and helpful book that follows the successful journey to fertility for fifteen couples. Each journey is unique but every woman – in her own way – had to learn to "let go". This is an invaluable resource for couples struggling to conceive.'

– Dr Judy Ford PhD, Geneticist and Fertility Advisor

'The stories in this wonderful book resonate strongly with the stories that my clients have shared with me over many years. Well done to Michaela Ryan for helping us feel the overwhelming emotions which can be experienced, as well as illustrating ways of coping with the downs and ups of infertility.'

– Miranda Montrone, Psychologist and Infertility Counsellor

'Honest, heart-warming and, at times, heart-wrenching – Michaela Ryan's anthology of personal anecdotes highlights the powerful experiences of couples who are trying to conceive. These stories show that its not enough to simply want a baby – many of these couples find that they have to sort out their own lives before they can take responsibility for creating another one. Told with sometimes painful insight mixed with delightful flashes of humour, these stories are illuminating and inspiring and will give great encouragement to everyone who wonders when their baby will come.'

– Karin Bishop, Editor, Essential, *The Sydney Morning Herald*

For Ted and Declan

Trying to Conceive

True stories of how couples overcame infertility

Edited by Michaela Ryan

Vermilion
LONDON

1 3 5 7 9 10 8 6 4 2

Published in 2009 by Vermilion, an imprint of Ebury Publishing
First published in Australia by Finch Publishing Pty Limited in 2008

Ebury Publishing is a Random House Group company

The Random House Group Limited Reg. No. 954009

Addresses for companies within the Random House Group can be found at
www.rbooks.co.uk

A CIP catalogue record for this book is available from the British Library

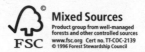

Mixed Sources
Product group from well-managed
forests and other controlled sources
www.fsc.org   Cert no. TT-COC-2139
© 1996 Forest Stewardship Council

The Random House Group Limited supports The Forest Stewardship
Council (FSC), the leading international forest certification organisation.
All our titles that are printed on Greenpeace approved FSC certified paper
carry the FSC logo. Our paper procurement policy can be found at
www.rbooks.co.uk/environment

Text designed and typeset by Pier Vido

Printed in the UK by CPI Mackays, Chatham, ME5 8TD

ISBN 978 0 09 192925 1

Copies are available at special rates for bulk orders. Contact the
sales development team on 020 7840 8487 for more information.

To buy books by your favourite authors and register for offers, visit www.rbooks.co.uk

Contents

Foreword

Michaela Ryan was inspired to write this book from her own experience of becoming pregnant after letting go of some emotional blocks she held, consciously and unconsciously.

Unfortunately, the emotional issues underlying conception have been largely ignored and sometimes disputed by physicians. From my own experience of working with infertile couples for more than 30 years, I have found that a successful conception often takes place once lifestyle and emotional changes take place. My own observations are supported by several recent studies that have shown improved pregnancy outcomes in women participating in stress reduction programs.

Couples experiencing fertility issues should carefully assess their environment and lifestyle. I like couples to check that their food is both nutritious and balanced, that their intake of water is high, alcohol is low, drugs are nil and smoking is nil, that they have no exposure to chemical toxins and that they exercise regularly. Ageing itself is a particular problem and needs special attention. There are a number of changes that occur physiologically at about age 36 which adversely affect fertility. These changes have a major effect on the critical 'oxygen carrying' functions of all cells, so older women need to optimise all aspects of their lifestyle.

In addition to these physical issues, I assess a couple's stress levels and their amount of sleep. Medical research clearly shows that, even if you are doing everything right in all aspects of health, you can quickly undo the good by having high levels of stress hormones in your body.

High levels of cortisol and related hormones can suppress ovulation, fertilisation and implantation. This will of course reduce the chances of becoming pregnant naturally. Even assisted conception can be more difficult for highly distressed women because, although ovulation can be induced artificially and fertilisation can be carried out in the laboratory, implantation has to occur naturally.

While stress hormones are often to blame, one study has shown that subjective emotional distress can impact on conception even in the absence of measurable changes in stress hormones. More research is required to fully understand this phenomenon.

This book discusses many of the stresses of modern life where the tendency to be driven by goals takes away from the peacefulness of just being. Stress can occur in the workplace, it can occur when you have unresolved issues about yourself as a future parent and it often occurs when you try to control life itself.

People respond differently to potentially stressful situations: one person's stress is another's stimulation. For example, one person may find a major change in work practices to be an exciting challenge while another may find the same situation highly confronting. Consequently, as stress is a very personal experience, there is no simple way of identifying situations that might contribute to infertility.

The internalised causes of stress are also different for each individual. However, the sort of stress that is harmful is often referred to as 'suppressed anger', otherwise known as 'keeping a lid on it'. Imagine keeping a lid pushed down on a boiling pot of water when the natural event would be for the lid to be lifted by the steam and the boiling water released all over the stove. It's not surprising that a number of people in this book conceived after experiencing a significant emotional outlet, such as having a good cry with a friend or talking with a therapist.

Emotional distress played a big part in the fertility issues experienced by the couples in this book. However, also present were problematic physical issues. Many of the stories involve women who delayed conception until their mid to late thirties. Many of the women (and men) describe having a career, with long hours and frequently long distances to travel. Some also had a social component to their work that involved too much alcohol. It's important to take a holistic approach to all of these influential factors.

I hope that many people will read Michaela's book before they find themselves overwhelmed by frustration and grief at not being able to conceive. If you, as a reader, have already moved along a more distressing track, hopefully you will be able to take guidance from these stories to restore your own personal peace.

Dr Judy Ford PhD
Geneticist and Fertility Advisor
www.ez-fertility.com.au

Introduction

I experienced some intense emotions and fears when my husband and I were trying to conceive. After a while, I instinctively knew that I was sabotaging the process. I believe I'm not just a body. I believe I'm made up of mind, body and spirit – and that each of these can affect the other. So eventually I decided to work my way out of my distress, and immediately I became pregnant.

I've since met many people with similar stories, so I decided to look further into this phenomenon. I came across many modern studies confirming the relationship between emotions and fertility (for more information, refer to the Editor's notes and Bibliography).

The stories in this book come from people who overcame infertility after shifting something on an emotional level. However, this book does not suggest that fertility problems should be addressed by dealing with emotional issues alone. It's often vital also to address problematic physical and lifestyle factors.

The thing is, your doctor can tell you all about the physical side of the equation. But there are not so many professionals or others addressing the emotional side.

One study has shown that the level of stress experienced by infertility patients is often similar to the stress endured by people suffering from serious illnesses such as cancer. When you consider these results, you can see why it's not very helpful to be told to 'relax' or to go on a holiday when you're having trouble conceiving.

As the stories in this book show, there can be many, many layers of emotional distress for a person with fertility problems. Sometimes the issues go right back to childhood. Sometimes they go to the core of a person's self-esteem. Sometimes they highlight a person's relationship problems. Sometimes they stem from a person's subconscious beliefs about parenthood, pregnancy or childbirth.

So let's say you're trying to conceive, and on some level you're aware that your emotions or thoughts or beliefs aren't helping. How can you work through these difficulties and bring yourself back to a state of being that's conducive to conception?

Each person's issues are different. And their physical responses to emotional distress are different. Therefore the solutions are diverse. Some people profiled in this book conceived after working through their issues by themselves – by making a conscious decision to create a new mindset. Others saw hypnotherapists, psychologists, healers. Some conceived once they brought the love back into their marriage. Others conceived when they let in the love and support of family members or friends.

My intention for gathering this collection of anecdotes was to present a smorgasbord of choices to people experiencing problems with conception. The ideas provided in these stories are far from exhaustive – but I hope they will at least get people thinking about the possibilities.

I don't specifically condone any of the techniques or treatments discussed in these pages. Like I said, everyone is different, so what works for one person won't necessarily work for someone else.

If you discover, as you read this book, that your own emotional state might be underlying your fertility issues, there is absolutely no need to feel any sense of blame or shame. You are not your emotions. You are not your stress. You are not your depression or anger or guilt or unhappiness. These are emotional states that can be resolved – often very quickly. Just as you would address a physical symptom in your reproductive organs, you can also address any emotional symptoms that show up while you are trying to conceive – and in doing so treat the whole person rather than just the body.

The people profiled in this book worked through their emotional issues to varying extents before conceiving. Those who had a really good look at their 'stuff' tended to have improved relationships, pregnancies and experiences of parenthood. So this isn't just about clearing up negative emotions in order to conceive – the benefits are far greater than that.

A small percentage of people do remain childless at the end of their fertility journey. For those who don't go on to have children, it's just as important to work through emotional distress. By nurturing yourself and your relationship you give yourself the best chance of creating a beautiful life – with or without biological children.

I hope you enjoy reading these stories, shared by myself and fourteen brave men and women who joined me in my mission to raise awareness and give people hope.

Just take from these pages what you need. If some information doesn't resonate with you, it's fine to ignore it. Only take on board the ideas that feel close to your own truth. Because it is in discovering your own truth that you will have access to all of the answers you need.

Michaela's story

IN MANY PARTS of THE WORLD, MEDICAL PROFESSIONALS INSIST THAT the twelve-month mark is some magical time when couples really need to get help conceiving. Looking back, the very idea of that twelve-month mark disempowered me. The closer I got to twelve months, the more I wondered whether there was some unassailable medical reason that I couldn't get pregnant.

Months rolled by. The more they added up, the more freaked out I became. Words like 'infertile' and 'adoption' began to enter my mind.

Was something wrong with me? Was something wrong with my husband? Because, surely, this was the most natural, easy thing for two people to do. You don't need a degree to do it. And obviously human beings have been doing it forever. It's something I just assumed, from the very earliest age when I was playing with my dolls, that I would do one day.

And for goodness sake, I'd been using contraception for so long and had been so paranoid about slipping up and accidentally getting pregnant that I just assumed that pregnancy was waiting to pounce on me at any possible opportunity.

'We're trying'

So let me take you back to the beginning of our journey, when my husband, Ted, and I made the decision to 'try'. I couldn't stand that word. I hated the idea that anyone who knew or suspected you were 'trying' might have a mental image of you and your partner, well, 'trying'. It sounded so shamelessly biological.

To be frank, we didn't really 'try' all that hard to begin with. I was only 27 and Ted was 29, so I thought it would happen naturally and easily. Dare I say it – I even thought it might be a bit romantic! So surely there wasn't really a need to do it *all the time*.

I promised myself I wouldn't let the process become mechanical or meaningless. I thought, *If it's meant to be, it will just happen without too much effort*. But as time went by, I realised that we might need to give Mother Nature a few more opportunities. And I realised that I needed to find out how my body actually worked.

My periods were so irregular that it was impossible to predict the timing of ovulation.

So after a few months I headed to the Internet to find out everything I needed to know about this topic.

There is a lot of stuff they don't teach you in school. Not surprisingly, 'how to get pregnant' falls into this category. So I actually found it quite informative when I did a Google search for keywords like 'ovulation', 'getting pregnant' and 'Billings method'.

By the time I learnt how to read my body a bit better, we were already six or seven months into the trying process.

Still more months passed by. More negative pregnancy tests.

I'd try to stay positive, but when the end of my cycle would come around, I couldn't help getting hopeful and excited, and then crashing with disappointment when the test was negative, or when my period arrived. At that point I'd become filled with doubt. And I'd think, *What if this never happens? What then?*

Several times I contemplated that I might never be a mother. I mightn't ever hold my baby in my arms and breastfeed. I mightn't ever be in a big family sitting around the dinner table laughing or arguing or celebrating someone's birthday.

When you're crying inside because you feel this lovely future is being snatched from you, there is only one thing that can make it worse. It's when someone says, 'So, do you think you and Ted will have kids soon?'

It's none of your damn business! I would scream on the inside, while politely deflecting the question.

Friends, strangers, colleagues … there seemed to be plenty of people with kids who wanted to give well-meaning advice about the road ahead, assuming Ted and I would be having kids some time soon. I was so consumed in my own anguish, I didn't even recognise their genuine attempt to help. Their words of wisdom just seemed clichéd to me. Sometimes even condescending.

Some people would tell me to enjoy my time without kids. They'd confide that parenthood wasn't actually all that great, telling me, 'It's the best thing you'll ever do, but the hardest thing you'll ever do.'

Again, I would smile politely, while my thoughts raged. Of course it's the best and hardest thing you'll ever do! I was under no illusion that parenthood would be like a nappy commercial. I could see that it would be hard work. But I felt ready for that chapter of my life. Ready for sleepless nights. Ready for stinky nappies and a crying baby. Ready for cracked nipples and stretch marks, and a messy house with toys all over the floor. I had the energy and the will to take all that on.

Then there was that smug, all-knowing comment: 'Nothing can prepare you for it. You just can't imagine what it's like until it happens to you.'

The immense love you feel for your children. The exhilaration you feel on the day your child is born. The exhaustion. The way your life is forever changed. Apparently these were concepts I had no way of understanding. These highs and lows were the exclusive domain of the parenthood club.

A lot's hanging on this

The longer we remained 'un-pregnant', I was forced to question something fundamental: my life's direction.

I'd reached a point where everything else was going well. I'd settled into my career. I'd settled into my marriage. But I had a strong feeling from somewhere deep within me that by being a mum I would derive a greater sense of meaning in my life. Just the thought of holding that dear little baby in my arms made me well up with unbelievable love. What a reason to get out of bed every morning!

Ted and I had prepared a space in our lives for a little one. For several little ones. We'd structured our careers, our finances and our travel plans around the idea that a child would be coming soon. Our lives – especially my life – were on hold.

I didn't want to become one of those women who was desperate about getting pregnant. I'd heard about people who were so stressed about conceiving that they repelled the very thing they wanted. But despite my best intentions, a good degree of desperation, and even obsession, crept in.

This is very embarrassing to admit, but I own a set of inspirational cards based on the Native American tradition. You ask a question and then you draw a card to find some advice, or an answer. I drew a few cards for fun, asking, 'Am I pregnant now?' or 'Will I get pregnant soon?' Then I started to draw cards all the time. And I'd get angry if the card didn't say what I was hoping to hear. I had this futile hope that I would one day pull out a card that said, 'Congratulations! You will fall pregnant imminently.' (Of course, I was willing to read between the lines for that message.)

Sadly, I became one of those women I didn't want to become. And I knew it. I knew also that my obsession was counterproductive. I knew I needed to chill out about it all.

Ironically, just thinking that I needed to relax actually stressed me out. How could I chill out when every month I clocked up made it more likely that I was infertile? How could I feel at peace when my life was on hold? How could I relax when everyone around me was finding conception such a walk in the park?

There were all these thoughts spinning around in my head, yet I had no-one to confide in other than my husband. I could have opened up to close friends, but for some reason I felt ashamed.

Eventually I shared the secret with my mum and my sister. I was pretty lucky, actually – neither of them offered any unwanted advice. They just provided a non-judgemental shoulder to cry on. It was cathartic having two extra people on my side providing encouragement and understanding. Best of all, I had a couple of people who I could laugh with about the whole situation.

> My desperation to become pregnant was only the tip of the iceberg.

My own worst enemy

Being as desperate as I was for a baby, I thought I was completely open and ready for motherhood. But I look back and realise that I was putting up a lot of resistance on a physical level, and on an emotional level. So it turns out I was my own worst enemy.

I was stressed out by a number of things. My desperation to become pregnant was only the tip of the iceberg.

For the first six months of this 'trying' game, I had a really stressful job. It was high pressure, long hours, and involved lots of driving. I was worrying about work when I wasn't there and, when I was there, I was powering through the day on a huge adrenaline rush. Even sleep wasn't giving me the rest I needed. I would dream about my work issues every night. Sometimes I'd gone through a day's work in my subconscious mind before I even woke up.

My body went into high-stress mode. I was losing weight and I had diarrhoea almost every day. I wasn't in a good state to be nurturing a little body and soul in my womb.

I actually had fleeting moments when I worried about what would happen if I did fall pregnant. There just wasn't the space or time for me to experience things like morning sickness, or take a day off to have a doctor's appointment. I even thought, *It's probably better if I don't get pregnant until this contract ends and I take a job with less stress.*

I eventually did get into an easier job and it did wonders for my health. I no longer took work home with me. I put some weight back on, and my digestive system came good.

When I took on the new job, I also had a huge desire to feel fit. So I joined a gym and started doing heaps of walking. I began to feel really good in my skin, for the first time in a while. So after about eight months of 'trying', my body was now ready. But what about my heart?

Looking back on my thoughts over that period, you would have to say I was like a yo-yo. I had so much longing for a baby, but to be completely honest, I couldn't help having the occasional thought of sheer terror at the thought of being a mum. I realise how strange that sounds – but I really was capable of wanting this thing so much, and yet at the same time being terrified by it.

One minute I would be writing in my journal about how much I couldn't wait to meet my baby; the next minute, I'd have a little freak-out, and purge it onto the pages of my trusty notebook.

I got nervous last night. I suddenly realised what is about to be ripped away from me – my beautiful, independent and deliciously selfish life. I have Ted all to myself and I love having him all to myself. All of his love and attention; all of his giggles and intimacy are shared with me – every ounce.

Now, when you arrive, Little One, we'll share each other with you. Our energy, our time will be stretched out between more human beings – as it should be. But I'll miss these days of Ted and me.

Don't worry, Little One, I already love you with all my heart. You will be the most amazing blessing in our lives. But for now, in this transition phase, as I contemplate my life being irreversibly turned on its head, I feel sad. I grieve. And a tiny part of me resents you for what you're about to take away from me.

What a cocktail of emotions! I found it so hard even to write the word 'resent'. I felt so incredibly guilty for feeling that way towards an innocent, 'un-conceived' baby. But the grief of losing my husband, which is how it felt at the time, was very real.

On top of that, I was so scared that my baby might experience some of the pain I'd known when I was growing up. I even questioned whether it was fair to bring a child into a world that had so much hardship.

> It has surprised me that in contemplating being a mum, I am being confronted with my own perceptions of motherhood. And the only example I had was full of struggle. Struggling to pay the rent and bills. Struggling to get enough sleep before a 5 a.m. shift.
>
> I don't want that for you. I want you to feel secure all the days of your life. I want you to appreciate the importance and value of money, without ever worrying about how your parents will pay the bills.
>
> I don't want you to know this pain. I will fight with every fibre of my being so that you never have to.

A couple of months on, I had another reason to freak out about having children: I spent more than 24 consecutive hours with other people's kids.

> I've been petrified lately.
>
> After two successive visits from mums with toddlers, I feel horrified by the exhaustion, the whingeing and the constant demands a small child brings.
>
> It repulsed me. And I've been confronted with a new set of questions, such as – should we travel overseas, and be young for a while longer? Should we just buy a house (which we're putting off because our income will drop if I have a baby)? Should we prolong our final days as a 'honeymoon-period' couple, enjoying our freedom and our sleep-ins?

I imagine now that my baby was sitting in the wings, waiting for an invitation. And with the mixed messages I was sending out, he or she must have been pretty confused! While I was holding a green light in one hand, I was putting up a stop sign in the other.

Over time I became aware that I was doing this yo-yo act. I knew instinctively that my attitude had to change before this baby could freely come into my life.

The big shift

My longing for a baby was causing me far too much grief. So I started to monitor my thoughts. I didn't allow myself the indulgence of any thoughts that dripped with desperation.

The keyword for me was 'patience'. Whenever a negative or desperate thought entered my mind, I took a deep breath and said the word 'patience'. I'd simultaneously feel the state of patience. It was a kind of peacefulness; a belief that everything was going to work out just perfectly.

I repeatedly told myself that my path was unfolding exactly as it should. I knew that I'd look back and realise it had all happened at the perfect time, for reasons I would only understand in retrospect. I genuinely decided I'd be accepting of whatever timeline, and whatever outcome, presented itself.

I stopped focusing on what I didn't have, and shifted my focus to the abundance I did have in my life. I reminded myself how lucky I was to have such a loving husband. Without him I wouldn't even have the luxury of contemplating motherhood.

I also got away from the idea that this baby would bring meaning to my life. I knew that was far too much of a burden for this other soul. It was my job to provide that sense of meaning for myself. I started to live my life as though it had meaning already. I started to plan the overseas trip I'd been pining for. I also started to properly appreciate the fun things Ted and I were doing as a couple.

For nearly a year, I'd restrained my alcohol intake just in case I was pregnant. But I decided just to have some fun and be myself, which meant having a few drinks and a lot of fun dancing when we'd go out occasionally with friends.

I looked at where my career path was going and started to plan some exciting projects for the medium and long term. That took away the feeling that my job was just a holding pattern until I became a mum.

I also read a beautiful book which helped me to feel really good about the idea of raising kids: *The Red Tent*, by Anita Diamant. The story depicts a family of women living in biblical times, helping each other to raise children. It paints a magical picture of what it means to be a woman. It taught me just how sacred it is to menstruate, to be pregnant, and to be a mother.

Baby news

I was in this new head space when my sister told me some news. Sitting on my bed chatting, I could see there was something she wasn't telling me. Eventually I dragged it out of her.

> It might seem weird, but in the same month I'd made this huge emotional shift, I finally became pregnant.

'I'm pregnant,' she said tentatively. Instead of looking excited, she looked guilty. She felt terrible telling me the news because it had happened straight-away for her.

I was nothing but thrilled! I threw my arms around her in excitement, and felt like busting open the champagne to celebrate.

It's a good thing we didn't open the champagne … little did I know, but at that moment I, too, had the very beginnings of a baby growing inside me. It might seem weird, but in the same month I'd made this huge emotional shift, I finally became pregnant.

Actually, I became pregnant exactly twelve months from the time we started to 'try'. I narrowly missed out on crossing that invisible, disempowering medical line that had been spooking me.

As I write these words, I have a healthy baby boy called Declan. He was born three weeks after his cousin – a baby girl called Tess. And just as I suspected, the timing was perfect. For so many reasons.

Suzanna's story

D AVE* AND I HAVE A FANTASTIC LIFE TOGETHER. WE LIVE ON THE water. Take our boat out every weekend. Our dream is to spend six months of every year in the Caribbean.

We're not sure how children fit into our vision. We'd like to have a family together. But it feels like we'd have to give up a lot. Dave is in his late thirties, so he's worried that he might be too old to be a dad and enjoy it properly. Nevertheless, we have to take the plunge at some stage because it's something we both want.

I'm convinced that I'll fall pregnant as soon as I go off the pill. I'm from a huge family. Surely Dave will just need to rub shoulders with me and we'll conceive. We're really going to do this! Here goes …

It's not happening straightaway. In fact, it's taking ages. That's beginning to stress me out. Is there something wrong with me? My periods only last for a couple of days. I'm not sure if I'm even ovulating.

It's just procreation. Why does it require us to work so hard?

Dave and I are feeling the pressure. We're arguing more than we used to. We argue about who left the toothpaste out. Who left the dishes in the sink. But that's not the real reason we're uptight. The tension is bubbling up because we want something so badly and it's not happening.

After about eighteen months I see a doctor. I have blood tests and the doctor assures me I'm ovulating on day 21 of my cycle. I have an investigative procedure called an HSG and I'm assured there are no physical reasons for our infertility. My first reaction is – yay! But then I feel even more frustrated than before. It sucks that there is no explanation for this.

The doctor asks if I am interested in assisted conception. No. I don't need help. Help is for wimps. I part ways with my doctor and continue to try the old-fashioned way.

You know what? The old-fashioned way is going from bad to worse. I remember when sex used to be fun and exciting. Now it's awful. A chore. And my attitude is not helping. I want this thing immediately, if not sooner. The pressure is getting to Dave, and sometimes he can't perform. We try to laugh our way through it but that doesn't always work. After each failure Dave feels less manly, which leads to more failure. I try not to be angry with him, but sometimes I can't help it.

My instincts tell me I'm not ovulating on day 21. I buy an ovulation kit to try to work it out. It tells me I'm not ovulating at all. Grrrr!

I take a new job, with medical insurance included in the package. Waiting for that to kick in, we decide to take a break from our conception efforts. It's nice to enjoy being with Dave without thinking about procreation the whole time.

When the break ends, it's back to the grindstone. My obsession returns. Dave's performance problems return. He even has his testosterone levels checked, but they're completely normal.

We've been flat out trying for nearly three years. Forget what I said about help being for wimps. I need some assistance here. What about alternative approaches? In my job as a sales rep, I often visit medical practices. Recently I saw a poster at one of the clinics, advertising acupuncture for fertility. Maybe that's worth a shot.

I have acupuncture weekly, and my next period is a nice, long ten-day job. Hooray!

My acupuncturist tells me about a psychotherapist who specialises in fertility issues. This lady helps people clear out any emotional blocks that might be preventing conception. Frankly, I'm a bit sceptical. But

I'm willing to try anything that might help, apart from conventional medical intervention.

Before my first appointment with the therapist, I rack my brains. Do I have any emotional blocks to conception? Yes I do. Dave and I have always had a fear of giving up our lifestyle. Maybe she can help me with that.

I meet my therapist, and very quickly she helps me realise that my issues around parenthood run a lot deeper than an impending change of lifestyle. It's time to revisit my childhood.

Going back in time

In my first couple of sessions with the therapist, I begin to share my childhood story. Out it all comes.

My dad had two wives before he married my mother. He had three children with those wives. Then there was my mum. She had four sons from a previous marriage. Then Mum and Dad got together and my mother's dream of having a daughter finally came true. (That's me!)

My brothers were still at home with us while I was little. They called my dad 'Pop' and he treated them as though they were his own children.

When I came into my mother's life she doted on me in every way. In all of my childhood memories, she's right there with me. Making me costumes for skating competitions. Helping me choose my outfit every morning. Putting my hair in a ponytail. I was always a little shy. When we'd go to a restaurant, I'd whisper my order to her and she'd tell the waiter what I wanted. My mum was my life, my whole world, my everything.

When I was nine years old, I found out my mother had breast cancer. She was ill for the next six months. She encouraged me to start being more independent, and I didn't like that one bit. One morning she refused to pick out an outfit with me. 'Go and choose it for yourself,' she said, ushering me away. I was furious. Later that day she was taken to hospital, and she passed away a week later.

I don't remember crying a lot after Mum died. But it hit me hard. Soon after, all of my brothers (except for the youngest, Johnny) moved out of home. It went from being a busy family household to a very quiet place. My mother's sisters stopped visiting us as frequently as they used to. I felt so alone in the world, and I missed my mum terribly.

My father remarried a year after Mum's passing. I couldn't stand the new woman in his life. To me, she seemed loud, abrasive and cold. Dad insisted that I call her Mum, but I refused. 'She's not my mum,' I'd scream. In time this lady nicknamed me 'the spoiled little bitch'.

This new woman brought one of her daughters to live with us, and my father began to treat his stepdaughter like royalty. It seemed that his affection gradually drifted away from my brothers and me. His 'new family' became the centre of his world.

Dining out was a whole new experience for me. I tried whispering my order to my dad once, but he brushed me off. 'Speak up! Tell the waiter what you want.'

That marriage only lasted for a couple of years. But Dad remarried again when I was thirteen. A new wife. A new stepmum. And no, I'm not calling her Mum either! A couple of new stepsiblings entered our house and the same pattern played out – Dad seemed to channel all of his love and attention to them.

In time my older brothers married. But sadly, three of them experienced the heartache of divorce first-hand.

As I share this story with my therapist, I realise how much anger I have been sitting on for my whole adult life. I am so very, very angry with my father.

A shock

I've barely begun therapy – I've only had two appointments – when I discover I am pregnant. For a whole week I float along on cloud nine.

Dave is cautious. He doesn't trust the home pregnancy test. 'Wait until the doctor confirms it,' he says.

Dave and I are against the idea of sharing our news with anyone before the end of the first trimester, but my therapist does a visualisation exercise that makes me change my mind on that issue. I visualise myself walking down a street and coming across a hotel which is all lit up – full of life and warmth and celebration. Across the road there is a dark, dim hotel with no-one in it. She suggests that for a baby in utero, the happy hotel is the place she or he wants to be. I decide that I agree. I want my baby to feel welcome, celebrated, acknowledged.

But before I have a chance to share the news with anyone, I head to the doctor's office for a urine test. I want to confirm the home pregnancy test results.

> Dave is cautious. He doesn't trust the home pregnancy test. 'Wait until the doctor confirms it,' he says.

'Honey, you're not pregnant. Whatever made you think you were?' says the doctor's assistant, who looks young enough to be at school. The test results are negative.

I'm not stupid, I think. *I had a positive test a week ago. I have pimples all over my chin. And my breasts are so tender I'd claw your eyes out if you touched them.*

Once I get over my anger at the twelve-year-old doctor's assistant, I'm beside myself with worry. I head off to a pathology lab to have a blood test done, since there is a chance that the urine test might have given a false negative. Now I'm howling uncontrollably in the pathology waiting room.

When it's my turn, a heavy lady with brown hair comes over and asks me, 'Have you ever had a blood test before?' Now I'm laughing. 'I'm not scared of having my blood drawn,' I assure her. When she hears about my situation, she rings the doctor to make sure my results can be returned urgently.

At home that afternoon I start spotting.

The doctor rings up with the test results. 'You are pregnant,' she tells me. Normally that phone call would be the most exciting thing in the world. But I tell her that I'm now bleeding.

'Spotting is nothing to worry about, unless you see blood clots,' she tells me.

Within a few hours the blood clots appear. It's a horrifying sensation. *I'm going to lose this baby. After everything we've been through. We've worked so hard for this. No!*

I spend most of that afternoon and evening lying on the sofa, bawling. Dave sits with me, also in tears. Then he heads outside to sit on the deck and be alone. We go to bed at 8 p.m. and hold each other all night.

Dave shares the news with his family. But they're the only ones who know about the miscarriage. There is no-one in my family I want to share this with.

Four days after the miscarriage, Dave and I decide to buy a condo as an investment. We both have misgivings about the purchase but we're not communicating with each other properly. I'm not communicating with anyone, because I start crying every time I try to speak. We go ahead with the condo, purely because we're trying to distract ourselves from our grief.

Now we have a renovation to oversee.

More therapy

My therapist asks me if I still have reservations, on some level, about falling pregnant. The truth is, I do.

At her suggestion, Dave and I decide to have a farewell ceremony for our baby. We stand in our lounge room holding hands.

'We're sorry that we weren't more accepting when you tried to join us. But please come back to us soon. We will be more prepared next time.'

It doesn't take me long to realise why my upbringing might be affecting my fertility.

I remember that, at the age of nineteen, I promised myself I would never get married and have children. I didn't believe marriage worked. And I never wanted to drag kids through the pain of divorce and step-parents. I've held onto that belief in my subconscious for a long time. Even as I've tried to start my own family, part of me hasn't believed that it's safe to bring kids into the world.

Part of me has also been petrified that I might die young and abandon my own child. Just like my mother.

My therapist asks if I'd like to challenge these beliefs and fears, and I do. I realise that I am not my family. Just because everyone else has failed marriages it doesn't mean I will. Just because my mum died young it doesn't mean I will.

All of these worries have created a huge inner conflict for me over the past few years. It's been really distressing for me emotionally, even though I haven't always been conscious of it. As I start to undo the conflict, I feel so much better within myself, and much more excited about starting my own family.

I also uncover some surprising attitudes towards my body and my femininity. A lot of them can be traced back to the day I got my first period. It was about a year or two after Mum died, and I was still very young. I went downstairs and told my dad. He thought it was the biggest joke, and let out a great, big laugh. I was mortified. Embarrassed, I ran back up to my room, and felt totally alone. I wished my mum was there. And I wished that I'd never have to have a period again.

I must have wished pretty hard, because I didn't have another period for a whole year. And when it did return, it only ever lasted for a day or so. Sometimes it was just a bit of spotting, and that was it.

Now in my therapist's office, I do a role play to tell my dad how I wish he'd reacted that day. 'Dad, you should have taken the time to tell me how wonderful this was. That it is one of the many beautiful wonders of the

female body. You should have said, "You are a woman now and this is very special. How would you like to celebrate?"'

I have a lot of anger in me that needs to come out. Something that helps me is punching pillows in my therapist's office. I do that at home too. I pound those pillows and release a lifetime of anger into them.

I also write letters to my father and my aunts. These aren't the kind of letters you send. They're the kind you write and then destroy. You say everything you've ever wanted to say but haven't been able to. I express a lot of anger in those letters. I'm upset at Dad for everything. And I'm upset at my aunties for abandoning me after my mother died.

I feel like my brothers abandoned me too. I'm not angry with them. Just disappointed. But I punch the pillows in their honour nonetheless!

After expressing my hurt, I realise that no-one really abandoned me. That was just an exaggerated creation of my nine-year-old mind. And I realise that it's not too late to forge closer connections with my brothers now. I'm looking forward to being in contact with them more than I have been.

I still feel sad about one particular aunt who left my life after Mum died. But I'm not as angry with her as I used to be.

One day my therapist gets me to imagine I am in a conversation with my mum. What would I want to tell her? I miss you. I wish you didn't die so young. I wish you had been at my wedding. I missed you so much on that day, Mum. I wish you were still here to become a grandmother and be around my future family.

During and after that process, I feel a lot of sadness. I go through a sense of grieving that I've never had a chance to experience before now.

No more needles

I drop the acupuncture a couple of months into my psychotherapy. My acupuncturist changes premises and I don't find the new surroundings relaxing. But my periods remain regular: they tend to last three to five days. And I have been ovulating, according to a new contraption I've purchased. It's an 'ovulation watch' with a sensor on the back that tells me when I'm fertile.

So all is well physically.

Softening

Emotionally, I'm feeling better all the time. Even the simple fact of being here with my therapist, expressing my feelings and admitting that I have issues to look at, is a humbling experience. I've been playing the 'tough girl' for a long time. I was so independent that I moved out of home literally on my eighteenth birthday. My attitude was: 'Don't mess with me.' For a while I

> The therapy helps me see what's really happening – how much the desire to conceive has come between us.

considered a military career. And I immersed myself in tae kwon do. My softness came back a little when Dave and I got together. But now I feel like I'm uncovering this whole other dimension of myself; one that is gentle and feminine.

After a while, I even start to feel better about my dad. There is still some anger there. But for the first time ever, I can see that he did the best job he could.

My relationship with Dave is definitely improving. You could say that I'm softening towards him, too. The therapy helps me see what's really happening – how much the desire to conceive has come between us.

I take a step back and remember that I married Dave for a reason. Of all the guys I'd ever dated, Dave was the only one I knew I could be with forever. He was my brother Johnny's best friend. He was always the life of the party. When I was 25 I asked him to be my date at Johnny's wedding, and we kept hanging out from that day on. He was a stable point in my world – and he still is.

It isn't worth destroying this awesome relationship because we're having a hard time conceiving. That's not to say I ease off on the pressure to have sex. When the words 'most fertile' appear on the screen of my trusty ovulation watch, it's time to go!

Dave attends a few sessions with me and he addresses some of the issues that have been coming up for him. He still wonders whether he can be a good father at his age. The therapist asks him whether he'd like to challenge his ideas about age. Yes. He would. *I can be a good father at any age*, he decides. And he also realises that having a child doesn't mean our lifestyle will come to a crashing halt. We'll keep life exciting, and do lots of travelling and sailing, even home school our kids so we can spend six months of the year in the Caribbean like we've always wanted.

When Dave first starts therapy, he's a little defensive, as if the therapist and I are ganging up on him. But after a couple of sessions he starts to get a lot out of it. Best of all, we start to grow closer. Gradually it feels as though we're being more loving during intercourse. We're also holding hands more. Kissing more. Talking more. Being the team that we were before we started trying to conceive.

Dave's performance issues are gone.

I'm feeling calmer in my everyday life. I'm still desperate to have a baby, but I believe that it will happen in time.

There has been no defining moment during these past months when things changed. It just seems that everything I've done has combined to make a big difference.

The only thing that's not going well is the renovation. We're losing money on the condo. That was the worst decision we've ever made.

Fighting in the car

After six months of therapy, I feel ready to take the next step, especially since I'm now thirty-five. Dave agrees. So I go to my doctor and I'm prescribed the fertility drug, clomid, to give my ovulation a boost.

These new drugs are making me so moody! Dave and I are in the car, showing our niece around town. When he takes a wrong turn, holy hell! I unleash my wrath on him. We have the worst argument ever. It's not like me at all.

Within a few days I hear news that my father is in hospital with liver cancer. I feel terrible about the fact that I haven't spoken to him for the past four months. Dave and I immediately head off to be with him. Dad is seriously ill, and we're told he only has a few months to live. We're staying in his house. Because of my taking the clomid, we're supposed to have sex a few nights in a row. The timing couldn't be worse. We do what we have to, but it feels very strange.

Still at Dad's place, and I'm feeling nauseous. Dave says, 'I think it's time for a pregnancy test.' Surely the clomid can't have worked that quickly?

We do the pregnancy test at Dad's house on Friday morning. The results show up immediately. Positive. We're nervous, elated, scared, in disbelief – all at the same time. We decide to keep the news to ourselves that morning while it sinks in.

That afternoon Dad has an appointment with his oncologist to get his schedule for chemotherapy. Four of us get in the elevator to leave together – Dad, his wife, Dave and me. Dad looks so downcast. I decide this is the right moment to give some good news. 'Today we found out that I'm pregnant.'

He gives me a huge hug and begins to cry. His wife says, 'Oh, that's wonderful!' By the time we reach the ground floor, Dad, Dave and I are all in tears.

Dad is simultaneously happy and sad. Thrilled about our news, but sad that he mightn't live to meet this grandchild.

I visit the doctor and she confirms that I'm pregnant. Several weeks pregnant. In other words, I was taking clomid after the fact. What I'd thought was my last period was just a bit of spotting that must have taken place as the embryo implanted. My first concern is: *Oh, my God! What has the clomid done to the baby?* The doctor assures me the baby will be okay.

At least there is an explanation for those outrageous mood swings that had us arguing in the car!

The happy hotel

Finally pregnant, I feel more determined than ever: I continue to work with my therapist so that I can have a healthy, happy pregnancy.

At the twenty-week scan, we find out the baby's sex. I give Dad a call to let him know we'll be having a baby girl called Victoria. They may never meet in person, but Dad is definitely in the warm and cheerful hotel, celebrating Victoria's life.

My dad passes away when I'm five months' pregnant. I feel so guilty that I didn't speak to him in the lead-up to his diagnosis. But compared to the way our relationship used to be, you'd have to say that we made our peace before his death.

I desperately wish my dad had lived to see Victoria at least once.

Happy baby

Our baby girl enters the world safe and sound four months later. Having her in our lives is just awesome. It's better than I could have imagined. She's a really happy baby – and only cries when she needs something. In fact, we made up a song in her honour that goes: 'Are you hungry? Are you sleepy? Did you poop?'

Victoria really loves her daddy. She's now nine months old, and he loves picking her up and dropping her on the sofa. She laughs hysterically, jumps down off the couch and crawls to him to do it again. This sometimes goes on for 30 minutes or more.

The therapy and acupuncture created the conditions in my mind and body – and in my relationship – that made it possible for me to finally have a baby. But it did a lot more than that. It helped me come to terms with my mother's death in a new way, and it helped me to connect with her again, in spirit. It brought me closer to my father in his dying days.

And it brought me closer to my brothers. They're a much bigger part of my life now than they've ever been. Victoria has a bunch of gorgeous uncles looking out for her. And she has a mummy who's carrying around a lot less emotional baggage than she used to.

I'm now experiencing a sense of 'family' that I haven't had since the age of nine. It's not just from having my own child, it also comes from restoring connections with the family from which I came.

Real names were replaced with pseudonyms in this story.

Rebecca's story

3

A T NINETEEN WEEKS, our BABY APPEARED ON THE ultrasound screen. He'd grown a lot since the first scan. 'Oh, look at his little legs!' I said. 'And you can see the heart.'

The image disappeared as the doctor put the ultrasound probe down.

'There's a problem here. We can't fix it today. But it's to do with the baby's heart,' he told us.

'No, no, no, no, no! What are you talking about?' I said.

A sense of shock covered us like a fog, and we didn't take in much from that moment on. Our baby probably wasn't going to make it. That much we understood.

We saw a diagnostic specialist a few days later. He spent 45 minutes doing an ultrasound and mapping out the baby's heart.

'There are only three spaces,' I said. That's when I realised our baby was missing a ventricle in his heart.

The doctor explained that there probably wasn't anything they could do. Even with surgery, they couldn't offer us a positive outcome.

Over the next day or so, an unbearable decision lay in front of us.

'I think we have to let him go,' I said to Nigel. He felt the same way.

I didn't think it was fair to let this little guy suffer. It wasn't fair to let him be born at full term, just to be ripped out and connected to a bypass machine before he was even disconnected from me. And I couldn't let the surgeons practise on my baby.

This little boy was never meant to be a baby crawling around in the world. He was just meant to be our baby whom we loved.

Although bringing the pregnancy to a premature end, I still had to go through labour and delivery.

I remember packing to go to hospital. I realised that this was the bag I should have been filling with baby things in preparation for a normal labour. Instead, I was putting a whole lot of shit in a bag, all the while carrying this empty, empty feeling inside me.

Nigel drove me to the hospital. I sat in the back seat of the car with my mum. With her arms around me, I cried and cried.

Going through that labour was one of the most difficult times of my life. But I can now look back and see so much beauty. My family and Nigel's family were all there, sharing food off my meal tray and chatting in between my contractions. There was a real togetherness.

At one stage, a nun joined me at my bedside and offered some words of wisdom.

'Life is like a tapestry,' she told me. 'Sometimes all you can see are the knots on the back. But eventually something happens that makes you view it in a different way, and you see the beautiful picture on the other side.

'The thing is, the tapestry is always beautiful. It's just that you can't always see the side which is beautiful.'

I knew she was right. But I still couldn't see anything but the knots in my situation.

Baby Max was delivered after fourteen hours, with no life in him. As his body emerged, there was this huge sense of peace – like a presence in the room.

'He's here,' I said, amazed.

Nigel, Mum and the midwives all had tears rolling down their faces. Every single person in the room could feel that same palpable presence and sense of calm.

Grieving

We had a small funeral for Max. He was laid to rest in a tiny white coffin carried by his two grandfathers.

I visited Max's grave regularly in the months that followed, not really coming to terms with my shock and grief. Nigel came with me sometimes. But usually it was just me. Nigel seemed to be getting on with his life while I was engulfed in grief.

The idea of having another child terrified me. I never wanted to expose myself to the potential for this much pain ever again. I was so afraid to have sex, because of what it might lead to.

After about six months we decided to move to the country for some dirt therapy. We wanted to get back to nature, have some chickens in our backyard and enjoy the mountain views. The process of moving house helped me take my mind off things for a short while.

All settled in, I suddenly found myself with nothing to do, other than my work as a nurse. Nigel often worked long hours, leaving me plenty of time alone with my thoughts. Sometimes when he'd arrive home I'd be totally worked up, ready to pick a fight with him.

I felt so angry with him for being so calm; so middle-of-the-road. Thankfully, I recalled the words of a midwife at Max's delivery. She told me that couples commonly break up following the loss of a child. 'If you want to stay together, you're going to have to accept that he will grieve very differently from you,' she warned me.

I had no idea what Nigel was really going through. In actual fact, he was on the brink of falling apart. Seeing how much I was struggling, he didn't want to burden me with his grief. So he chose to process it internally. Catching up with friends and getting on with life was his way of 'being strong'. He was trying to convey the message that he was okay, and I could lean on him as much as I needed to. His intentions were admirable, but unfortunately they backfired. All I wanted was to hear how much he was hurting, so that I didn't feel so alone.

I loved our country home. But living there, my grief and depression only worsened. My thoughts became suicidal at times. Mostly they were just thoughts, nothing I would have acted on. I didn't want to leave Nigel and all the other people I loved in the same state of grief that had overwhelmed me. But one day I seriously contemplated driving off the side of the road. It terrified me, and made me realise how unwell I was.

I talked it through with Nigel and created a safety net of a few people who knew how black it seemed to me. They were people who weren't so scared by the blackness that they would drag me out of it before I was ready. But they knew to keep an eye on me.

Eventually I saw the need to escape my own thoughts. So I started studying midwifery. I'd been moved by the role the midwives had played at Max's birth. Perhaps it was an area in which I could make a difference? I was in total denial about my underlying motivation for studying midwifery: I wanted to be around babies. I wanted to see first-hand that healthy babies are born all the time.

Nigel felt ready to try for another baby before I did. He kept reminding me, 'Isn't this what we want? To be parents?' It was what I wanted, but it still felt too scary.

A huge conflict was welling up inside me. On the one hand, I was fearful of being pregnant. But more and more, I found myself longing for a baby. I thought it might fill a huge void in my life. Yet that desire for another baby made me feel quite guilty – I didn't want to devalue Max's life by 'replacing' him.

It wasn't long after we arrived at our new home that we tentatively started to 'try' again. But I was still very fearful. It was more a case of being less careful than we had been, rather than actively trying.

Several months passed, and I kept thinking of something my GP had told me. 'You mightn't ever get over this fear of falling pregnant, so don't put it off for so long that you miss out.' Eventually I decided he was right.

So after six months of 'not being careful', we started to try to conceive in a serious way. I was terrified, but willing.

My willingness was driven by a primitive feeling from deep within that I needed to mother a child. And in some ways, I still believed that a baby might help fix my pain.

Trying again

In no time, my thoughts were completely preoccupied with conceiving. It was a welcome distraction from my grief – although that wasn't a conscious thing.

I read everything I could get my hands on, and I came to understand the science of conception extremely well. That compounded my sense of frustration because nothing was working.

> ... the worst question of all was: 'Do you think you're a bit stressed?'

I was doing all the things that are supposed to help you fall pregnant. Naturopathy, the Billings method, improving my fitness, new hobbies – I even bought a dog. Still, nothing.

It felt so cruel that my cycle stretched out beyond the standard 28 days, giving me false hope every time. I got so annoyed with my body. One day I spoke to it in my journal, writing:

> My period is due tomorrow. I want it to either come on time, or not come at all. It's not fair for it to be late, if I'm not pregnant. So that is the challenge, Body. On time, or not at all. So there!

I was sick of people telling me they knew this would be my year – that they knew someone who lost a baby just like Max, who went on to have ten healthy children. That we should take a holiday. Aaaagh! *Fuck off!*

I hated it when people asked if I was trying. It was worse when someone asked if I was pregnant yet. But the worst question of all was: 'Do you think you're a bit stressed?'

I knew my distress must be impacting on my body, but telling myself to stop feeling like that made it so much worse.

My workplace was a breeding ground for 'well-meaning' questions and comments. In the end I felt so confronted by it all, I resigned. I started to do agency nursing, to be anonymous for a while.

More and more I started to wonder about my alternatives. I felt a little relieved at the idea of adopting. Maybe it would be a less risky way to create a family? I'd never have to face the loss of a baby or the prospect of physical abnormalities. But I felt nothing but despair as I searched through websites, reading about the hurdles we'd have to overcome to adopt a child.

Slowly I opened myself to the possibility of fertility treatment. It briefly occurred to me that my relationship with Nigel might be too strained to cope with the process of in vitro fertilisation.

Things weren't great between us. I was giving Nigel a hard time over the smallest things. 'I can't believe you would drink all the milk and not bother to buy a new carton.' 'How could you go and get yourself a glass of water and not offer me one?'

Whenever we had a conversation, I'd pretend to listen, but I was always busy with my own thoughts. They were only ever about the one thing. Conception, conception, conception.

Intellectually, I knew I should be addressing the cracks in our relationship. But I didn't do anything about it. I couldn't see it at the time, but I was too consumed by my own distress to really care about him.

The metamorphosis

Eventually a friend recommended a natural fertility clinic – a place which took a holistic approach to a couple's lifestyle and diet. I liked the idea, but I thought I might have to drag Nigel there. He's a very concrete, sceptical guy. I assumed he would have a lot of doubts.

Turns out I was wrong. The woman at the clinic gave us lots of research-based information to take home. Nigel read it all, and it made sense to him. We could both see how important it was to get our bodies in the best possible shape so that the sperm and egg could develop properly and have the best possible chance of sticking together and making a healthy baby. Nigel came on board as a willing participant, my partner in this mission.

We reduced our exposure to certain toxins, chemicals and radiation. We took some horrible potions, swallowed loads of supplements and improved our diets. We began eating lots of organic food. Nigel's commitment impressed me no end. He even gave up beer!

Nigel enjoyed the compliments on his new physique – he lost 8 kilograms. I lost 5 kilograms, so my body image improved a lot too. I felt so physically able!

Although we'd started this natural fertility approach, we were keen to find out more about IVF. We went to an obstetrician to find out whether we would be likely candidates for the process. He organised some tests for Nigel and me. The upshot – neither of us had a glaring physical problem. Nigel had a few abnormal-looking sperm, but the number of healthy sperm was well above average. I had some endometriosis. But it wasn't significant enough to be an issue, and they managed to clear it away.

The obstetrician showed us some statistics about our chances of falling pregnant naturally, given how long we'd been trying, and our ages. I was 29 at the time, and Nigel was 31, and the stats looked pretty grim. That night Nigel said to me, 'If our chances are so low, surely getting some help is a good idea'. I agreed. But because of the cost of IVF, we decided to put it off for a month or two.

As we continued our natural fertility approach, life started to feel easier. I felt really in tune with my body, and with my soul as well.

I went back to a psychologist who I'd seen a few times after losing Max. During a session with her, I realised that I didn't really want to continue my midwifery studies. I wanted to get on with what I did best, which was giving people tons of care in the emergency department. Working and studying, I'd put myself under enormous pressure. It felt so liberating to drop all of that.

I returned to a regular job as an emergency nurse. I was ready to be part of a team again. I got lots of great feedback in my new role, and felt really capable.

I decided to stop beating myself up about my emotional turmoil. For so long I'd been wishing my grief and anger and frustration would just go away. Now I realised I had to experience these feelings. Until I gave myself permission to do that, and let that journey take as long as it needed, I was never going to be all right.

I had always thought other people weren't comfortable with my grief. Actually it was me who hadn't been comfortable with it. I'd been ashamed, and felt as though I was keeping some dark secrets. But as I started to feel okay about my stuff, I began to communicate more freely. I opened up in a new way with Nigel, and with a few close friends.

I also spoke really candidly with my colleagues about the upcoming IVF procedures. My fertility issues became a tea-room discussion topic. Because I was so relaxed about it, so was everyone else around me. I felt really nurtured by my new group of workmates.

My relationship with Nigel was also improving. I wrote in my journal:

> I feel so much better. I don't want to be angry or upset at Nigel any more. I'm trying to focus on him, put myself aside and be interested in things beyond myself. I love him. I need to show him that.

One day we were sitting on our deck together, overlooking the mountains, and I told him how much happier I was.

'I can definitely see that,' he told me. 'And it feels as though you're remembering why we wanted to have a family in the first place. It's because we really like each other, and we want to create a life together.'

All I could do was nod. We were in total agreement.

From then on, there was no sense of having a baby in order to fill a gap in our lives.

IVF

After trying for eighteen months, we got the IVF ball rolling.

I tolerated the scans and the drugs really well. I didn't have big mood swings, and I stayed really positive.

My colleagues were fantastic. They administered the hormone injections I needed for IVF, and helped me stay light-hearted about it all. I'd read somewhere that the follicle-stimulating hormone is produced from Chinese hamster ovary cells. So we did this 'Chinese hamster face' at work all the time to make each other laugh. (Nowadays the FSH is a synthetic hormone, so I think the Chinese hamsters are off the hook.)

Going into my first stimulated cycle, I felt excited. The staff were sensitive, and referred to us by our names. But I still felt a little vulnerable. It was as though I was outside of myself as I observed this scientific process happening around me and to me.

The day before my first egg collection was the second anniversary of Max's birth. Nigel and I went to the cemetery together and went through our 'memory box'. We looked over the cards people had given us, official documentation about Max's birth, and a photo of me when I was pregnant with him. It was really therapeutic, and we felt full of love for Max. I felt such strength from my bond with Nigel that day.

> I tolerated the scans and the drugs really well. I didn't have big mood swings, and I stayed really positive.

My first egg collection was extraordinary: thirty of them were harvested; eighteen embryos came from those.

Intellectually I knew it might take a while, but I couldn't help thinking maybe it would only take one go. So when my period arrived a couple of weeks after the first implantation, I felt knocked out.

I rang my nurse at the IVF clinic and grumbled, 'I just got my period.'

'That's really crappy,' she said. 'If you like, you can come in for a blood test, and once we've confirmed you're not pregnant, you could start the next cycle right away.'

'All right, let's do it,' I said.

A few days later, I sat with the clinic's counsellor. I communicated all of my emotions. I felt let down. Pissed off. Frustrated. I'd lost faith in my own intuition.

'Everything you're feeling about this process is normal,' she reassured me.

That was all I needed to hear. I remembered what I'd discovered for myself in recent months – the worst thing you can do is to tell yourself not to feel something.

During the second cycle, I still had a sense of vulnerability during the procedures. I wasn't yet accustomed to this surreal scientific world.

When that second attempt failed, I again felt bloody disappointed. But I resigned myself to the fact that it might take ages. I started wondering what I'd do down the track: *How will I know when it's time to give up?*

During the third cycle, I cottoned on to the fact that my luteal phase (the time between ovulation and menstruation) was quite short. I had a chat to my nurse and my specialist, and they agreed that next time I should try some medication that would encourage the lining of my uterus to stay receptive to the embryo for a bit longer.

I headed into my fourth cycle with renewed energy. I wasn't just going through the motions any more. It felt like I was in the driver's seat, customising this process to my own body.

I wrote in my journal:

> I feel a strength of spirit and an endurance, and I don't think it is just me getting on with it. I think Max is with me. And I think God is showing the way.

I felt as though I'd learnt so many lessons since losing Max, and I was finally ready for a positive outcome, whenever that might happen.

A couple of weeks after the procedure, I had some spotting. *It's all over,* I thought. Just like the previous two cycles.

Then the spotting stopped. *This is strange. The only other time this happened, I was pregnant with Max,* I thought.

I did a pregnancy test and there was a faint positive result. I was desperate to believe that I might be pregnant. But at the same time, I was terrified to believe it, in case I was mistaken.

I organised to have a blood test at 8 a.m. the next morning.

I wouldn't get the results until 12.30 p.m. Nigel was at work, so I camped out at a friend's house for the morning. I pretended to listen to what she was saying but I was constantly trying to sneak another look at the clock.

At 1 p.m., having received no word, I couldn't stand it any longer. I caved in and rang the nurse. 'Are the blood tests back?' I asked, desperate and excited.

'Not yet.'

Nigel rang me on my friend's landline to see what was happening. 'Nothing yet,' I told him. Then my mobile phone started to ring.

'What are you doing in November?' the nurse asked me.

'I don't know. What am I doing in November?'

'Would you like to have a baby?' she asked.

I screamed, 'Oh my God!'

My friend was so excited for me. There were sobs and hugs, and I quickly rang Nigel to tell him the news.

As I drove home, I don't think the wheels of my car were even on the ground. It was like being in a hovercraft!

The road to 'mumhood'

I was anxious around the time of each scan, and I contemplated the possibility of this baby having abnormalities. But for some reason I knew he or she would be born at full term.

With conception out of my mind, I discovered a whole other side to life – the side that had nothing to do with babies! Suddenly I was listening to what was happening in other people's lives.

Nigel was really cautious during the pregnancy. 'Do you want to feel the baby kicking?' I'd ask him. But he didn't want to. He wasn't going to get attached until this baby was born.

I remember visiting Max's grave when I was heavily pregnant. I wanted to be thrilled about this new baby, but it felt like I was leaving Max behind. Life was taking a new turn and soon I'd have a little person in my life consuming all of my attention. *I wonder how long it's going to be until I come back here.*

When I was 38 weeks' pregnant, I started to feel some niggles in my lower abdomen. They niggled away for a day and a half, and I had no idea whether it was the start of labour or not. In any case, I decided I should beautify myself for my hospital experience! So I went in for a bikini and eyebrow wax. I sat on a towel, just in case my membranes ruptured. Halfway through the waxing, I said to the beautician, 'I think you're going to have to do that a lot quicker. I'm going into labour.'

By the time I was at the cash register, waiting for my credit card to be handed back to me, I was bent over with my head on the counter.

I had a beautiful birth, and felt very in tune. When our son, Nicholas, was placed in my arms I kept saying, over and over, 'Hello, little baby. We've been waiting to meet you.' Finally free to express his feelings, Nigel was glassy eyed, and completely amazed by the whole thing. In no time, he was an expert on nappy changes and blanket wrapping.

I felt completely spun out by how amazing it was to have this perfect little baby in my life. But I was also very anxious. I waited for the weather report every afternoon, using the overnight temperature prediction to calculate the number of blankets Nicholas would need.

No problem!

Our return to IVF happened as soon as I'd weaned Nicholas off breastfeeding and had my first period. Nigel and I were in the most terrific frame of mind about it all. We knew exactly what we were signing up for. IVF. Pregnancy. Birth. Interrupted sleep. Lots of joy. Lots of work. No problem. *Bring it on. And if the IVF takes a while, so be it.*

Back I went to implant another frozen embryo, feeling very matter-of-fact about it all.

A couple of weeks later, some spotting came. And then a day later, it stopped. *Surely not. It can't be that simple.*

I was having a massage that day, and I arrived early at my appointment. Early enough to run into a nearby pharmacy and grab a pregnancy test. I used it in the

> We knew exactly what we were signing up for. IVF. Pregnancy. Birth. Interrupted sleep. Lots of joy. Lots of work.

toilet at the day spa. It was there that I discovered I really was pregnant. I went out and told the masseuse.

'I just found out I'm pregnant.'

'Oh, that's great. Congratulations,' she said.

'No, I mean, I literally just found out, in your bathroom!'

Surprise, surprise

Nearly two years later, Nigel and I were heading to a tropical island for a family holiday with our two sons, Nicholas and Seamus. I was still breastfeeding Seamus, but my periods had come back. That got me thinking about when I should head back for another shot at IVF. I was keen to do it right away, but Nigel suggested we should wait until after our holiday.

'Let's just mellow out and enjoy being a couple and a family,' he said.

It was very unlike me to be so relaxed, but I agreed with him. You can't breastfeed while you're going through IVF, and I liked the idea of breastfeeding a bit longer.

My period was due the day we arrived on the island, so I'd packed my bag full of sanitary pads and tampons.

A few days into the holiday, my period still hadn't come. Every day I'd update Nigel. 'Still no period. Oh my God, just imagine …' And he'd tell me not to get ahead of myself. It was just so unlikely.

In the end, I couldn't contain my suspicions. I looked everywhere for a pregnancy test, but not a single shop stocked them.

I decided it would be okay to tell people who didn't matter. Lounging by the pool, I told some of the other resort guests that we'd just found out I was pregnant. I wanted to enjoy the fantasy. Since having Max, I believed that keeping a pregnancy top secret for the first twelve weeks wasn't fair to the baby.

At first it was painful to look back on the times I'd felt blissful with Max in my womb. The joy of feeling him move for the first time. The warmth I had felt as I rubbed my belly. But eventually I came to treasure those memories. They were the times when Max was with us.

When I was pregnant with Nicholas and Seamus, I'd told everyone right from the start. I wanted other people's prayers and hopes on my side. And sitting by the pool in our resort, I didn't want this to be any different … just in case.

After our return flight, we got home at 11 p.m. I went straight to an old pregnancy test in the bathroom drawer, and had a shower while I was waiting for the result. When I hopped out, there were two lines. I very calmly took the test into Nigel and held it up.

'So, what are you doing in April?' I smiled.

Our tapestry

Now we have our two boys, and a wide-eyed baby girl called Lucy.

I'll always see Max as one of the greatest blessings in my life. He laid the groundwork for Nigel and I to become the best parents we could be. As a couple, we relate to each other so differently now.

And I relate to everyone in my life differently, because of the huge changes I went through.

Sometimes I take the children to visit the cemetery where Max is buried. They know he's their brother, and they call his grave 'the remembering place'.

I often think of the nun who sat with me during my labour with Max.

She was right about that tapestry. All we could see were the knots and mess for a bloody long time. But eventually we came to see something far more beautiful, and far more amazing.

Mark's story

I REMEMBER THE EXACT TIME – 10 P.M. I WAS DRIVING HOME FROM dinner at my parents' place, with my wife, Charlotte*, dozing in the passenger seat beside me. The radio hummed with love songs and dedications. The cruise control was set at 100 kilometres an hour as we headed down the freeway. I had no idea that my life was about to change dramatically.

A teenage boy ran out in front of us. I didn't even have time to hit the brakes. He hurtled into our windscreen. Charlotte woke, and for a split second he looked straight into her eyes. They were the last moments of that boy's life. The image of his face stayed with Charlotte and me for a long time.

We both felt devastated by the accident. But it also jolted us out of the way we'd been looking at life.

As newlyweds, we'd been enjoying our time with dual incomes and basically having a lot of fun. We thought we'd have kids one day, but we weren't ready to give up our lifestyle just yet.

Within 24 hours of the accident, Charlotte told me she was ready to have kids. Life was short and precious. She wanted to leave a legacy to the world – and our children would be a big part of our legacy.

Charlotte had already been off the pill for about six months, but her cycle hadn't returned. Life without periods had been a novelty for her. But now we wanted to have a baby, she started to worry about it.

Another six months passed, and her cycle still didn't come back. She booked in to see an obstetrician who specialised in fertility issues. We then realised that nothing happens quickly in the fertility process. We had a ten-week wait for the appointment.

> All of these processes were happening to Charlotte, so that put me in a support role by default. I felt like my job was to stay as upbeat as possible for her.

From the moment we saw the obstetrician, a sense of urgency kicked in. It felt like we'd lost more than a year, just mucking around. It dawned on us that I was 33 and Charlotte was in her late twenties, and we had a job to do, as soon as possible. The obstetrician was part of our team now, and we were going to work together to get Charlotte pregnant.

The problem seemed to be that Charlotte wasn't ovulating. She began a series of fertility treatments that would last for eighteen months. Hormone tablets, dietary changes, internal examinations. All in an effort to kick-start her cycle. More time and patience were needed, as we waited to see whether we'd have success with each new thing we tried.

All of these processes were happening to Charlotte, so that put me in a support role by default. I felt like my job was to stay as upbeat as possible for her.

The hormones sometimes made her moody on top of the frustration she was already feeling. At times I'd cop it over trivial issues. 'Why didn't you think to clean the benchtops/pick up your clothes/do the ironing/offer to help me with the shopping?' They were all things I was happy to do. Previously she would have just asked for help and I would have been on to it. But now there was a new kind of tension in these everyday encounters.

I tried to roll with the punches, making allowances for her because of the hormones. But sometimes I would have had enough, and I would bark back. After those occasional verbal stoushes, we'd both go and sulk at different ends of the house for a while. But we always made up by the time we went to bed. My nan's advice about relationships often came back to me: 'Never let the sun set on an argument.'

Although it was my job to ride out the bumps with Charlotte, there were some things I could never understand – especially when it came to the things her body was going through. She shared a lot of those details with her mum, and that mother–daughter relationship made up for the areas where I couldn't empathise even if I had wanted to.

The sex

With fertility treatments on the go, suddenly there was a set of rules governing our sex life. Because of the fertility drugs, we were required to have sex three nights in a row at a certain time of Charlotte's cycle. I remember one night when we both got home from work feeling exhausted.

'Should we just leave it till tomorrow?' Charlotte suggested.

'No. We better do this,' I said. 'I'll do you a deal. It's 10.38 p.m. now. It will be lights out at 10.43.'

'Cool, you've got a deal,' she said.

True to my word, at 10.43 p.m. we were done. We laughed and pumped the air with our fists in mock celebration.

> ... the reality was a clinical sex life, which often felt like hard work. There wasn't all that much loving in it.

Thankfully we were able to keep moments like that light-hearted. But the reality was a clinical sex life, which often felt like hard work. There wasn't all that much loving in it.

Hard to stay upbeat

When a fair bit of time had passed, I realised we were dealing with something big. It wasn't going to be fixed overnight – or possibly ever. The thing that hit in really deep for me was seeing how much my wife wanted to have kids. Of course, I wanted the same thing, but I didn't think it would be fair for me to express that. I wanted to make sure that Charlotte never felt any pressure from me whatsoever.

I always assured her that her health was my main priority. 'If, at the end of this, we don't have kids, that's cool,' I told her. 'As long as you come through it healthy, we'll be okay.'

I loved going to see my mate's kids playing football and that sort of thing. But I was always careful not to get too attached to the idea of being a dad. I put a big shield up in front of myself to guard against my own potential disappointment. Above all, I didn't want any paternal instincts to bubble up and become obvious to Charlotte. That was the last thing she should be worrying about.

Pushing down my desire to be a dad became harder as more of our friends started to have babies. We'd shared our twenty-first birthdays. Then our engagements and weddings. Now it was the era of the newborn babies. With each new birth, I felt more and more pressure. It felt a bit like being in a race.

We often went to visit our friends' new babies in hospital. *I wonder what it would be like if it were Charlotte and me sitting on the bed next to our newborn, with people visiting us?* When I'd see Charlotte cuddling a baby, my breath would catch for a moment. *She seems so genuinely happy for our friends. But I wonder what she's really feeling deep down.*

Occasionally we'd get home from those visits and our own reality would hit us hard – especially Charlotte. But we were determined not to alienate ourselves from those friends. 'If we don't have our own, we're going to adopt one of our mate's kids as a surrogate,' I'd say.

IVF

None of the treatments improved Charlotte's situation. In vitro fertilisation was our next option.

Before our obstetrician could refer us to the IVF specialist, I had to produce a specimen. They wanted to know what they would be dealing with on both sides.

I have to admit that, the first time I had to provide a sample, I looked at the tiny plastic jar and thought: *Is this going to be big enough?* Like many men before me, and many more to follow in this strange world, I would soon learn that a small jar is all that is required.

Sitting in the obstetrician's office, we were given my test results. 'Unfortunately your sperm count is very low,' he said. The tears started flowing for both of us. I was absolutely gutted. I don't like losing, and I don't like being told I can't do something. On top of all the obstacles we'd already faced, this felt like the final nail in the coffin.

I kept wondering why my results were so bad. I wondered if it had something to do with an undescended testicle I'd had as a kid. Or maybe I'd done something wrong as an adult? Had I incurred any damage through long distance running?

> I was absolutely gutted. I don't like losing, and I don't like being told I can't do something.

The state of a man's semen can change in the course of a week, so I did another test a week later to double-check. This time the results were even worse. The obstetrician told us that even if everything had been okay with Charlotte we would have needed IVF to overcome my issues.

After my initial disappointment, I actually felt relieved. It wasn't all about Charlotte any more. I could share the responsibility with her.

The good news was that, in theory, my problem could easily be overcome using IVF technology: under a microscope they could fish out the healthy sperm.

Counselling

Our IVF doctor suggested that we seek out any alternative medicine which might complement the IVF process. So in the two months leading up to the first cycle, we went to see a homeopath recommended by Charlotte's mum. Thankfully, she was happy to work alongside Western medicine, offering us remedies that would support us before and during IVF.

The homeopath also provided us with counselling. I had a few tears in her office on a couple of occasions when we told her what the last two years had been like. Before then, I don't think Charlotte had understood the impact it had had on me.

I was feeling frustrated and powerless. If I could have put myself in Charlotte's position, and been the one to take hormones and go through all those procedures, I would have done that. If I could have handed over every dollar I had in order to change things, I would have done so. But it felt like there was nothing I could do to make the situation right.

The counselling definitely allowed Charlotte to see that the pressure had mounted in me.

She was surprised when I explained that I hadn't wanted to express my feelings before now, because that might have put pressure on her. 'I thought maybe you didn't really want to have kids,' she said.

She was absolutely rapt when she realised I wanted kids as much as she did. A weight was lifted. Beyond this point, our teamwork went to a much higher level.

We had a couple of friends who had been through IVF, and they offered to act as our mentors. I couldn't recommend that highly enough – their support and advice was really helpful.

They told us we needed to have a Plan B; we couldn't pin all of our hopes on IVF. We ran with that. We decided to see the IVF as an experiment. It mightn't work out, and if that were the case, we'd create a different kind of life for ourselves. (I imagined in this alternative life I would be driving an Audi TT, but we didn't go into too many specifics.)

Other friends and family members offered support in their own way. 'Stay positive' was the most clichéd and annoying thing anyone said. It got to Charlotte more than it did to me. Given her heightened emotions and all those hormones in her system, such comments were like holding a red rag to a bull.

I liked it when friends showed an interest and really listened to our thoughts and experiences. It was great when we could share stories and have a laugh about it all. When people said things like 'I hope everything goes well for you', that was perfect.

We commenced our first cycle of IVF, which would last 60 days from start to finish. I was on edge the whole time, because we needed to stick to a rigorous schedule of events. One tiny stuff-up and it would be game over – another two months before we could start again. Since the timing was critical, I kept setting the alarm on my phone and I called Charlotte to remind her to take tablets, inject herself and inhale a nasal spray. I could hardly think of anything else.

> Afterwards, I carefully put my sample jar in a polystyrene box. I didn't want to spill a drop.

The big day

The day of the egg pick-up arrived. I was allowed into the theatre while they removed Charlotte's eggs. Under sedation, she squirmed and grimaced. I remember the doctor saying, 'Can someone hold her still?' It was traumatic watching her go through that, and not being able to do anything about it.

With Charlotte in recovery, I was told to go upstairs to provide a semen sample. Just before I headed off, Charlotte joked that my part was ridiculously easy compared to everything she'd just been through. And it was.

A nurse showed me into 'the room'. It was like a mini lounge room, with a TV, a couch and some magazines.

Knowing there was a waiting room, predominantly full of women, on the other side of the wall, there was definitely some performance pressure. I felt a bit embarrassed, but there was no time for airs and graces. I was part of the IVF program. I had a job to do. A deep breath and away you go.

Afterwards, I carefully put my sample jar in a polystyrene box. I didn't want to spill a drop. It felt like liquid gold! *Hopefully between all you boys there's a good one in there somewhere*, I thought.

I just had to get across that waiting room and hand it over to a member of staff. *How do I play this?* I wondered. *Should I leave in a hurry? Or play it cool?*

I probably looked like a little kid walking out of there with a guilty smirk on my face. Everyone in that room knew exactly what I'd been up to for the last ten minutes.

Forty-eight hours later, the embryo was implanted. Now we had a fourteen-day wait ahead of us. If Charlotte got her period in that time, all bets were off. But if she got to day fourteen, a blood test would tell us if she was pregnant or not.

We counted down the days, and the tension built up with every 24 hours that passed. I would sometimes look at Charlotte and think: *Shouldn't she be sitting with her legs up in the air? Would it help if she crossed her legs?*

Trying to stay relaxed, we spent a lot of time with family and close friends. We all had a good laugh as I recounted my tale of carrying the polystyrene box through the waiting room. And Charlotte had some hilarious 'party stories' about her experiences too. Our friends couldn't believe how much fun we were able to have with the whole thing.

Day fourteen

As day fourteen came around, we were quietly confident, but still not wanting to get our hopes up.

Our 'IVF mentors' told us to plan something to do on the evening of the blood test. That night would be a screaming high or a screaming low, they told us. Either way, you want to have something planned to help you get through. So we organised to meet Charlotte's parents at a restaurant.

Charlotte had her blood test first thing in the morning, and was told to expect a phone call between 12 p.m. and 3 p.m. We decided that she would visit me in person once she knew the result, whether it was a win, lose or draw.

I had my phone by my side all day, and I was constantly checking to make sure the battery was full and the signal was strong.

When that phone call finally came through, I ran straight downstairs to meet Charlotte.

'I don't want to talk about it out in the open. Let's go for a coffee,' she suggested.

We held hands and went across the road to a café. It felt as though I was about to open a birthday present. But once a present's open, it's open. I wanted to savour those minutes before I knew for sure what Charlotte was going to say.

Sitting in the café, Charlotte really strung out the story. She had been waiting all afternoon without hearing from the nurse. At 2.50 p.m. she picked up the phone.

'I can't wait any longer,' she told the nurse.

'We're going through alphabetically,' the nurse explained. 'And we're nearly up to you. But I guess since we have you on the phone already, we can give you the result. Are you sitting down?'

Instantly, all of the subconscious pressure lifted off my shoulders. We were pregnant!

'Yes …'

'Yours has taken,' the nurse told her.

'Thank you. Thank you. Thank you.'

The nurse had been really happy to tell Charlotte this news, because she had just delivered a long list of disappointing results to other patients.

After everything Charlotte had put herself through for the last two and a half years, this was the best news we could ask for. It was an unbelievable feeling. Instantly, all of the subconscious pressure lifted off my shoulders. We were pregnant!

We felt a bit guilty as we thought of all of the other people who hadn't received good news that day. But we still felt an incredible excitement. I can only really compare it to the feeling of being newly engaged. We were a couple of jabber jaws. *We're going to be parents! Who should we tell first? How should we tell them?* A million thoughts ran through our minds. I felt like doing cartwheels.

So much for that Audi. Every day I head off to work in a car which I affectionately call the 'family truckster'.

That night, we arrived at the restaurant, as planned. My parents-in-law were sitting there nervously, not wanting to ask us about the results, but looking desperate to know. When we told them our news, it was one of the biggest moments of their life. Nothing can compare to the reaction of a close-knit family to news like that.

Charlotte's mum pulled a baby's rattle out of her handbag for us. A rattle for her first grandchild.

We decided to wait until the end of the first trimester before announcing the news to our friends. The next ten weeks went so slowly; I couldn't wait to scream it from the roof tops.

Becoming a dad

Witnessing my son's birth was overwhelming. It was the most amazing thing. Charlotte and I both cried when we first saw him.

On the one hand, being a father has really brought out a protective side of me. And on the other, it has helped me to soften.

With this little guy in my life, it feels like I have a new purpose. Someone who depends on me. I want to do the best job I possibly can in raising him.

So much for that Audi. Every day I head off to work in a car which I affectionately call the 'family truckster'.

Charlotte loves being a mum, and the three of us have been very contented in our first year as a family. We really have brought something special into the world, just as we envisaged after that car accident.

As if …

When Jack was eleven months old, Charlotte took him for a visit to the GP. The doctor enquired whether we would be having another baby.

'We think we'll go back and do IVF again at the end of the year,' she told him.

'Will you need IVF this time around?' he asked as he flicked through her history. 'Oh yeah, you're going back to IVF,' he concluded.

After having Jack, Charlotte's periods had returned to normal, but the doctor thought that the problem on my side of the fence would make a natural conception difficult.

> The next day, Charlotte woke up feeling as sick as a dog. We assumed it must be food poisoning.

A two-stripe surprise

The next day, Charlotte woke up feeling as sick as a dog. We assumed it must be food poisoning. But she happened to say, 'Do you think we should go and get a pregnancy test?'

'Can't hurt to have one in the cupboard,' I said. 'But as if we're going to be pregnant.'

We went down the street and bought a test, putting it aside while Charlotte spent the whole day lying on the couch and throwing up.

The next morning Charlotte went into the bathroom, and after a while I heard her say, 'You might want to come in here …'

I went in and she showed me the pregnancy test with two stripes on it.

'What does two stripes mean?' I asked her.

'It means I'm pregnant.'

'Well, you better get out the other test then,' I said. 'You couldn't be.'

She did another test. And the two stripes showed up again.

We wanted to get excited, but we still weren't convinced. So the next day Charlotte went back to see the GP. He assured her the tests wouldn't have given a false positive.

'But hang on, weren't we just saying a few days ago that you needed IVF?' he said, confused.

He was as surprised as we were.

> Only two things had changed since the time my sperm tests had come back with such poor results: my undies and my attitude.

Only two things had changed since the time my sperm tests had come back with such poor results: my undies and my attitude.

I'd started wearing boxers instead of underpants. That was the only thing that was different on a physical level.

The other difference was my mindset. With Jack in our lives, we had nothing to prove any more. The weight of expectation was gone. The performance pressure was nowhere to be seen. Conception was hardly on our minds. We thought we'd return to IVF later on, but we were so grateful to have Jack in our lives that we knew it would be okay if it didn't work out this time.

Life was busy, and my job was stressful, but on the whole we were very content with our lot.

Oh, and there was one other thing that was different. The day we conceived this second baby, the sex was the most loving and fun sex we'd had since Jack had been born. We had laughed and enjoyed ourselves heaps. Nothing clinical about it. So even though I was surprised that Charlotte fell pregnant, when I thought back to the day of the conception, I wasn't that surprised.

The blessing of Charlotte becoming pregnant with a second child without having to go through the rigours of IVF is fantastic. Now we're counting down the weeks until our second baby's birth!

What a journey this has been. The key to it all has been our strength as a couple. By keeping our relationship the priority, it made the process so much easier than it might otherwise have been. Keeping our sense of humour was a big part of that. It was also really important that neither of us ever put any blame on the other.

I'm in such a privileged position, because I can now say that Jack and our next baby are the most amazing things we have done as a couple. Nothing can take that away from us.

* *Real names were replaced with pseudonyms in this story.*

Deb's story

A T HE IVF clinic, I'VE COME TO KNOW THE DAY SURGERY NURSES by name. We swap the names of books we're reading. I always bring one to read after a procedure. They know to leave me alone when I return from theatre, confident I know the drill.

My world consists of endlessly intrusive scans, drugs, consultations and procedures. I'm fed up with the prodding, the loss of dignity, the constant invasion of privacy.

Sometimes I feel that I'm part of a production line. I almost expect them to finish with me and yell out, 'Okay, next!'

Every couple of months we have a fresh shot. Then an excruciating wait until the day we do the pregnancy test.

Testing day is a ritual. I do a home pregnancy test first thing in the morning, and then place it on Keith's bedside table. We cuddle in bed until it's time to look at the result. Sometimes Keith tells me it's negative. Other times he just turns around and hugs me without saying anything.

Those days are the hardest. Sometimes I need to stay home from work to grieve. Other times I think, *To hell with it*. I buy a packet of cigarettes, then plug myself back into my daily routine and wait for the next cycle to begin.

The disappointments come one after the other, like rounds in a boxing ring. Every time, I dig deep, somehow finding the determination to press on. I remind myself, *I'm just one step closer to having a baby. Next time it could be positive.*

We've had two positive results already. Twice, we've had our hopes raised sky-high. The first time we had a positive test in front of us, we looked at it in disbelief. Disbelief made way for dizzy excitement. For the next couple of days, we kept looking at each other, knowing we had this little secret we couldn't share with anyone else. Then I started to bleed.

I went in for an internal scan. Keith was there, holding my hand. Our specialist confirmed what I'd been fearing anyway. There was no heartbeat.

'I'm so sorry, Deb. You're having a miscarriage,' he told me.

I looked at Keith and said, 'We'll be all right.'

Don't cry. Be brave.

Our specialist hugged me as I left. The feelings welled up and so did the tears. A big breath, and out we walked to the car park. It wasn't until we were tucked away inside our car that I lost it. Keith held me while I sobbed.

Within a month of the miscarriage, three other people in my office told me they were pregnant. *Maybe all the babies are going to everyone else and I'm going to miss out,* I thought. Then I would remind myself, *Just because someone else is pregnant, it doesn't affect my chances of conceiving.*

Eventually I came to see that miscarriage as just another hurdle. I moved on. So did Keith. We were one step closer.

The second time we had a positive test we were just as excited. But we were sceptical. We tried not to talk about the pregnancy too much in case we jinxed it. Ten weeks in, I started bleeding. Another miscarriage. The doubts crept on in. *Am I capable of carrying a child in me? Is this a sign that I should discontinue IVF? Maybe my body isn't ready. Maybe I'm not ready.*

Keith wanted to be strong and supportive, so he hid his pain from me. I did lots of talking and crying, and he sat with me through it all. When I asked how he was going, he reassured me, 'I'll be fine. It's you I'm worried about.' I had no idea how overwhelmed he was feeling. No idea that he was breaking down in tears in the car park at work.

For all those years, Keith had been keeping our struggles to himself. But after that second miscarriage, he was pretty raw. One day his boss – an old friend – mentioned a couple who had miscarried. It was impossible for Keith to hide his emotions. It all came out. The IVF, the miscarriages, the grief. His boss was completely understanding. He told Keith he could take as much time off for appointments as he needed. He was so relieved he didn't have to carry this secret around any more.

Conception is my life

Disappointment is an emotion I seem to handle okay. But a much bigger emotion has engulfed me over time, and I don't know what to do with it. Desperation. It has been nearly four years of back-to-back IVF. I am eating, sleeping and breathing *conception*.

I'm doing all the right things. Yoga and meditation. Eating lots of free-range chicken and red meat (yuk). Plenty of organic fresh fruit and vegetables. No wine, caffeine, chocolate … and (almost) no cigarettes.

My body had some problems at the outset. Polycystic ovaries. Endometriosis. Some potentially cancerous cervical cells. But our specialist assures me that none of these issues should prevent me from conceiving on IVF.

So, when is this going to happen?

I've done the career path, Keith's successfully worked his way towards achieving his career dreams, we're building a wonderful new house. We just want a baby to complete the next chapter. Is that too much to ask?

It's hard seeing three year olds strapped in their strollers with mothers ignoring their cries. *Let me have that child*, I think. *I'll take great care of him, spoil him with everything, smother him with love.*

My whole pay packet goes towards our IVF treatments, but I don't care. I'll do whatever it takes and pay whatever it costs.

My mother has told me I'm obsessed, that I need to let go. Of course I'm obsessed. It feels like this is my life's ambition. How could I let it go? What would I do then?

All of this is hard enough to deal with. But on top of that there are the mood swings. The fertility drugs make me feel out of control. I'm like a rubber band about to snap. I cry over insignificant events, like dropping mail on the floor. Then I get so mad, and I don't even know why. I can experience an onslaught of completely different emotions, all within five minutes.

I'm too overwhelmed and over-drugged to be bothered with details. Thankfully, Keith has a brilliant memory for dates. He takes in everything our specialist says, and reminds me about my drugs, scans and surgeries. He's always there to pick me up after my procedures. He always remains positive. He's quietly confident that one day we are going to be parents.

But we are not happy any more. All we seem to talk about is IVF. Keith thinks my obsession is dangerously affecting my physical and emotional wellbeing. He thinks I need a break in order to regain some control of myself. But I'm like a runaway train – I can't stop.

What else can I do?

I'm willing to try anything that might help us to have a baby. I'm already doing everything I can to make this work on a physical level. But I'm starting to realise this isn't just about me having injections and treatments and sprays. Keith is right, I have to start looking after myself emotionally.

The first thing I want to do is get some understanding about the things that went awry in my childhood. Ever since I decided to have kids, all of these unhappy memories have been right in my face. Mum and Dad arguing. Dad coming home drunk and being violent.

Mum took us to live with our grandparents when I was nine. Dad visited us there for a few years but one day he stopped showing up. *He doesn't give a shit about me*, I thought.

I've heard about people repeating the same mistakes their parents made. It scares the hell out of me. I'm not at all confident in my ability to be a good mother. And I want to do something about that.

I share some of my worries with Mum. She casually suggests that it might help to get in touch with Dad again. At first I'm taken aback. I haven't seen this man for 23 years.

If I see him, and hear him apologise, I wonder if I might be able to heal some of the anxiety, the anger, the rejection, the pain. They're all sitting here, wrapped up tightly in a box. I'm holding all of that negativity in my body somewhere, and blaming Dad for the lot. I'd really love to let it go.

My brother calls me with some news. Dad has been in hospital with a brain aneurism. He nearly died. This is the kick I need.

I press the phone to my ear. My stomach is churning and I can actually hear my own heart beating.

'Gosh, it's so good to hear from you!' my dad's voice booms.

'Dad, I don't have any happy memories of you,' I tell him. 'I thought it was time we started creating some.'

> I'm holding all of that negativity in my body somewhere, and blaming Dad for the lot. I'd really love to let it go.

Now that we're in contact, I don't seem to need an apology. That's just as well, because he hasn't offered one. But one day he explains why he stopped visiting us. He says he didn't want to disrupt our lives any more. I believe him. A huge weight lifts. My confidence returns.

The next step

I've started to receive acupuncture from a lady I briefly saw when I started IVF. She's showing me how to assist myself in becoming pregnant, like tweaking my nipples to get everything stimulated! I'm enjoying the light-heartedness of it, compared to the brutality of IVF. She's also helping me to become more in tune with my physical being. Her treatments 'heat up' my uterus, and increase the flow of energy to that area. I'm really seeing how important it is to take a holistic approach to conception. It's not just tablets and injections that my body needs.

I feel calm and meditative when I leave my acupuncture appointments. It makes me realise how tightly wound up I've been.

I've been so involved in my own stuff that I haven't noticed how much I've changed these past five years. Keith and I are only just becoming aware of it. We're almost in shock now that we can see what we've created.

I've stopped playing all the sports I love. I've dropped my hobbies. Bit by bit I've unplugged from my life – and I've unplugged from myself. Keith even says, 'You're not the same girl I married.'

He's not himself either. He's been hiding away with me in this private world. We reached a point when it got too difficult to turn up to dinner parties and pretend everything was fine. It seemed easier to shut ourselves away.

'Do you want to take a break from IVF?' Keith asks, again.

'No,' I say, 'I don't need a break from IVF. I need a break from myself.'

I feel battle weary. But that's not because of the IVF. It's because I've spent so long feeling desperate and negative and focused on nothing but babies. I want to step out of my skin for a while and feel like someone else. Or the girl I used to be.

I'm taking six months off work. I'm going to continue my yoga and acupuncture, and write a list of all the things I would do if only I had more time. I've always loved making things, knitting, cooking, gardening, painting, reading … It's time to throw myself back into the things I love.

My beautiful break

I'm living the life of a busy housewife. No stress. No anxiety. No time constraints or routines. Keith has never been so well fed in his life. I'm cooking up a storm for dinner, and sending him off to work laden with homemade treats.

I've organised the pantry and restocked the freezer. I've picked up books I've been meaning to read for years.

Keith and I are reconnecting with our friends, one by one. I literally go through our address book and say, 'Oh, that's right ... now let's give these guys a call.'

Finally we've stopped thinking, *We'll be happy when IVF is over and we're parents.* We're enjoying life and the people who are around us now.

I can now see that, without kids, there are other things I could commit my time to. There are so many places to explore, so many things to learn in our journey through life, so many more people to meet.

I've even started to tell close friends that if I'm not pregnant at the end of this six-month break from work, then that will be it. We'll sell the house and go overseas. Will I really carry that out? Maybe I could just extend it for another six months ... We'll see.

A different result

It's a few months into my break and I've had my twenty-third IVF cycle. (I've actually lost count, but it's something like that.) Time for our old ritual.

We wait a few minutes, just like every other time we've done this. Keith rolls over and hands me the test. *It'll be negative,* I tell myself. But it's not. I burst into tears. He bursts into tears. No words will come out. We just look at each other and hug for an eternity.

We don't know what to do with ourselves. It has been such a long time since we have had a positive result. 'Let's not get our hopes up,' we tell each other. 'Let's wait until we do the proper blood test.' But then every ten minutes we're cuddling each other again and getting so excited. I've been taking such good care of myself maybe it really will happen this time?

The blood tests confirm that I'm really and truly pregnant. I just have to hold my breath and get through the first trimester, then the second and the third. I'm not taking anything for granted.

Sometimes I lie on the couch and rub my tummy and cry because I can't believe this is happening. I don't care about the morning sickness. Absolutely nothing can mar the joy of this pregnancy.

At fourteen weeks, I'm back at work. I feel renewed. An old and tired chapter has finished. The next chapter will have new characters, new beginnings, all unknown and mysterious.

I'm a mum

I started this whole process when I was 30. Now, at the age of 36, I've become a mum.

My daughter's birth was the most joyful occasion. Our specialist was there to deliver her by c-section. He had been through every step of the way with us, and it felt so perfect to have him there to witness that miraculous day. The moment she was born, I felt such gratitude towards him. I reached past the little barrier they put up in the middle of my torso, put my hand on his arm and said, 'Thank you,' with tears in my eyes. The whole room froze for a moment. I'd contaminated the surgeon! He had to be re-scrubbed before he could continue.

Lily is just so fabulous. It's taking a while to become accustomed to her behaviours, although we were fairly prepared for the sleep interruptions, the dinner interruptions, and all the other little interruptions. We embrace them because she is here – finally.

Keith's a natural at parenting. Lily's often unsettled between 2 a.m. and 5 a.m. When I've fed her and done everything I can, Keith takes over. Down they head to the lounge room where he puts on some music and rocks her in his arms for as long as it takes. I love seeing this big, masculine man with this tiny, vulnerable girl.

Keith and I feel so much closer. 'Let's not take any of these moments for granted,' we tell each other. We've learnt through IVF that every moment is meaningful, an opportunity for something. We're having the greatest time. Maybe we could do this again …

Our second

My daughter is eighteen months old and I'm thinking it would be great to have a sister or a brother for her.

'Do you want to go again?' I ask Keith.

'You're not ready,' he says.

I know what I'd be in for with IVF. I think I can handle it. But Keith has some pretty vivid memories of my emotional distress. He is worried about seeing me go through that again. He can see I'm stressed out at the moment. Our finances are drained and I've had to go back to work part-time. I hate leaving my little girl in daycare so I literally run from the train station to the childcare centre so she doesn't have to be there a minute too long. I've also been helping Mum find a nursing home for Grandma. I'm exhausted actually.

The thing is, I'm 37 now. Hello! The body clock is ticking. Surely it won't be that hard returning to IVF. We already have our beautiful daughter, so the pressure will be off this time. If it doesn't work, it doesn't work.

Keith reluctantly agrees, and we head back into IVF.

It's a joy to see our specialist again, and to know that he'll be with us for every step of this new journey.

Drugs, appointments, procedures. It's a familiar environment. But I was wrong. It's not going to be any easier. Now that I'm here, I really want this baby. I don't feel the same level of desperation, but that huge determination and drive has come flooding back.

Everyone is telling me it will happen quickly this time, and that has put a lot of pressure on me. What if it doesn't?

The first cycle is followed by a negative test. Normally I'd need some time to let that sink in, to process my grief. But life is so busy now. I don't have time for that. I'm still at work, and when I'm not there, I'm taking care of the constant needs of a toddler.

Keith knows I'm not coping that well. I can't do this without his total commitment, so I'm going to wait until he's behind me. I need a few months to convince him that I'm genuinely ready.

Here we go again

A few months have passed and Keith and I are on the same page again. I've decided to recreate the circumstances that helped me fall pregnant with Lily. I've taken six months off work, and I'm seeing my acupuncturist again. It's not quite the same blissful, stress-free existence that I created a few years back. But it's definitely an improvement.

I'm not feeling the same level of excitement I did when I attempted IVF a few months ago. I'm still determined to make it work, but I'm over the whole IVF experience. It's mundane and I'm sick of doing it. I just want the result without all the drama.

All the people involved are thinking positively and encouraging me, and I just want to tell them to keep it real for me. I know the drill. It could take months, years to conceive and I'm prepared for it.

It happened!

After two more cycles of IVF, I've fallen pregnant! No more treatments. What a relief. Keith is also relieved.

We're still reserved about the result, and we discuss the possibility of the big 'M'. I tell Keith, 'If I miscarry, I'm not going back into IVF.' I just couldn't cope. I've done my time and this is it. He tells me I'd better put my feet up for the next nine months in that case.

In the late stages of labour, I've been rushed in for an emergency c-section. It's all happening. Medical staff are frantically doing their work. Keith is holding my hand, feeling very anxious about whether our obstetrician will arrive on time.

In the next breath, I have a perfect baby girl placed on my chest.

In hospital, I indulge myself more than I did last time. I limit the number of visitors and just enjoy being together with this little one. Lily and Daddy visit every day. Lily can't take her eyes off Alayna.

End of an era

It's time for Alayna's six-week check-up. But this doesn't feel like a regular doctor's appointment. I've brought my whole family in, for a very special reason.

Nine years ago Keith and I walked into this office as a couple. Now here we are: a family of four. I feel like our specialist is a friend. I've watched him get married and have his own children.

I've written him a card which says, 'You have been part of a life-changing experience for us and helped us to fulfil our dreams, not only once, but twice.'

As I leave the clinic, I start sobbing. It feels strange and sad to be ending our relationship with our specialist just like that.

I'm also incredibly relieved. This is all over. I don't have to put myself through this any more. I can completely unwind from those harrowing years on the road to parenthood.

Today

Our IVF years were tough. But so much good has come from them. These days I love providing support and understanding to my friends who are going through the same experience. When they get a negative result, I always remind them that they're one step closer.

Looking at my two beautiful angels, I know that long, hard road was worth it. Every minute I spend with them is a gift.

Alicia's story

I'LL NEVER FORGET THE WORDS THAT CAME OUT OF THE anaesthetist's mouth. It was awful enough being in there, about to undergo a termination. And then he casually said to me, 'So you want to get rid of it, do you?'

'Actually, it has trisomy eighteen,' I told him.

The foetus I was carrying had a chromosomal defect, making it incompatible with life. You should have seen the look of horror as the doctor registered what I had said, and quickly apologised.

This was my first pregnancy – a beautiful stage of life I'd expected would happen smoothly and easily. It had only taken four months to conceive. This baby was planned, and it was wanted in the world by my husband, Bill*, and me.

When we found out about the trisomy eighteen, we'd been given two choices – neither of them good. We could terminate the pregnancy now. Or we could let the baby grow. But it would either be stillborn or die soon after its birth. We decided on a termination.

The whole procedure was very clinical. Bright hospital lights. Medical staff moving about with purpose. Equipment beeping around me. But 'clinical' was good. I didn't want anyone fussing around me making it an even bigger issue.

Afterwards, we found out that the baby had been a boy. That made it more difficult; more real.

Four months later, I fell pregnant with Baby Number Two. Sure we'd had a rough trot the first time around, but chances were everything would be fine this time. Then, at eleven weeks I started to bleed. To allay any concerns we organised an ultrasound for the following day.

I can only describe the appointment as surreal. An image appeared on the screen and straightaway we knew something was wrong. The foetus was tiny. We looked to the doctor for an explanation. His face was ashen. 'I'm so sorry. The foetus has died,' he reluctantly told us.

Soon after, the bleeding got heavier. Then came the curette. A cold, clinical procedure to remove the foetus. The nurses made the whole experience bearable, treating me with kindness and compassion as if a full-term baby had died.

A few more months passed before I fell pregnant again. But this little soul let go at six weeks. I miscarried naturally, just before Christmas. Crap, what a year.

I remember feeling pretty numb that Christmas. Defeated and empty.

Spotlight on our relationship

Before our struggle to conceive, Bill and I had busy jobs and active social lives. We lived together as husband and wife, but we didn't really give each other the time that any relationship deserves. However, when we lost those three babies, our reality changed. It was no longer just about ticking the box and having a baby. We had to start spending time together. We had to start talking. There were some big questions we had to ask each other. What did we both think of terminating a pregnancy? Was there something wrong with us? With me? Should we change our obstetrician? Was this our future; should we adopt?

I can see now that our relationship wasn't really strong enough for us to become parents back then. That twelve-month period brought a lot of lessons for us as a couple – but there were plenty more to come.

Anger

The numbness I experienced that Christmas eventually turned into anger. Frustrated, I wondered, *How is it that thousands of babies are born every day?* I was angry at us for not being able to get it right. I'm not overly controlling, but I like to be able to do things; to make a difference with things. When it came to having a child, we couldn't do that.

We were surrounded by a lot of people who were getting pregnant and having kids. Eventually we chose to disassociate ourselves from babies and birthday parties. We couldn't help it. Rightly or wrongly, it was a way of protecting ourselves.

Our friends and family noticed our distance. Most of them tiptoed around us when required and gave us endless love, support and understanding, even when we would brush it aside. Friends who had babies were considerate of our feelings, at a time when we should have been celebrating in the joy of their new arrivals. Sadly, though, in distancing ourselves we ended up losing a couple of friends.

Change of path

I knew something massive had to change in my life in order for me to sustain a pregnancy. Clearly, whatever I'd done so far wasn't working.

Everyone was telling me, 'Alicia you're working too hard. Stress doesn't help when you're pregnant.' So I decided to remove the one thing in my life that everyone else believed was at fault – my job.

Quitting my job was like ticking another box. *Everything should be fine now. My body can rest. My mind can clear.*

I switched my obstetrician for a high-risk specialist. What a gem that man was. He ran a number of blood tests and discovered that blood clotting may have affected my pregnancies. He put me on a small daily dose of aspirin to thin the blood. To try and counter any further chromosomal problems, he increased my daily folate intake. So with these two things I was armed and ready. Well, so I thought.

I was doing everything I thought I should – all my energy was now going into getting pregnant. I was off work, I was exercising more and I was tracking my cycle. But nothing happened! Each month we hoped. Each month we waited. Each month disappeared with no result.

I had read somewhere that naturopathy can sometimes help with fertility issues. I decided to give it a try. I'd always believed that traditional and alternative medicine could complement each other, but in this instance it wasn't the case. The advice from the naturopath contradicted my obstetrician's advice. I ended up confused and upset. While I wanted to do anything I could to get pregnant, too much advice proved destructive and demoralising. Needless to say, my naturopath visits were short-lived.

So much for quitting work to clear my mind! My emotional distress gradually grew worse. My self-esteem was at rock bottom. I hadn't been able to hold on to a pregnancy. My cycle had blown out to 38 days. And now I couldn't even fall pregnant. *Clearly there is something wrong with me*, I believed.

I felt guilty that I wasn't earning money. *I don't deserve to be off work*, I thought. *Only mums with babies deserve to be at home.* When I would run into people who were stay-at-home mums, I found myself justifying how I was spending my days.

I really struggled with my lack of direction. I needed something else to focus on. So I decided to try volunteer work with a charity for women who had lost babies through stillbirth and miscarriage. After two days, I realised I couldn't do it. They had me sifting through entries for a 'cutest baby competition'. The worst thing I could have done!

Bill was initially relieved when I quit work. But as the emotional roller coaster worsened, he was forced to come along for the ride. The whole idea of my taking 'time off' was working against both of us.

At times we felt really angry and didn't want to be with each other. (Having sex was a chore at those times.) We even had days when we decided we shouldn't be together and that, clearly, not being able to have a baby was a 'sign'. We wondered whether we would be good parents anyway.

On our more positive days, we remembered how lucky we were just to have each other.

> Somehow we found our way back to the roots of our relationship. We remembered why we had got married in the first place.

Back to work

I'd had enough of treading water. I needed to return to my career for the sake of my sanity. I landed myself a great full-time job – certainly one that I could throw myself into and forget my own thoughts. By now, those thoughts were full of frustration, anger, blame and doubt.

Let's have a breather, we decided. It had been two very stressful years and we needed space from the whole baby thing. Bill was sad that we wouldn't be trying for the next six months, but he knew I needed a break.

During that period we cultivated a much greater respect for each other. We started to do things like going out for long lunches at wineries and going away for weekends – stuff that people with kids can't do. We were forced to sit across the table from one another and talk. It's incredible how you can forget to do that when you're running a house and living your life. Somehow we found our way back to the roots of our relationship. We remembered why we had got married in the first place. We'd lost that along the way and taken each other for granted.

Whatever happens, we'll have each other – we took great comfort from that. And we started to make plans for our life together. We decided that if I wasn't pregnant within a year, we would head overseas for a working holiday. It was an exciting option and we really sank our teeth into it.

Trying again

By the end of our six-month break, our relationship was going well. My self-esteem had improved quite a lot by going back to work. It felt good to be doing something productive.

Another really subtle thing happened at that time which lightened my spirit. The whole time we'd been trying to conceive, I'd had this underlying wish to give Mum and Dad a new grandchild. I had felt disappointed for them that it mightn't happen. But one day my mum said, 'When you go overseas ...' She knew that an overseas adventure was our Plan B. So with those words, I knew she had accepted that we may never have kids. That was really reassuring for me.

Something else which really helped was seeing a hypnotherapist. I'd never done anything like that before. I was seeing a homeopath about some headaches I was experiencing, and he suggested I see the hypnotherapist who worked in the same centre, as he thought it might help me to address some of the anger and fear I was feeling.

The hypnotherapy was a good outlet. It was another way for me to repair the damage that had been done to my self-esteem. It allowed me to talk to my subconscious – instilling the ideas that I was a good person, that I deserved to be happy and that I deserved to be pregnant.

A lot of negative emotions had built up over the past few years. I went back in time – even to when I was quite young – and revisited situations that had carried similar emotions. I took my adult self into those scenarios and reassured the younger me that everything was going to turn out okay, and that I was a good person. In doing that, I healed the negative emotions associated with those past events, and then carried that same reassurance forward to my current situation.

During the hypnotherapy sessions, I also used visualisation techniques, such as putting all of my fears and anger on a boat and watching it sail away. I actually started to use this sort of visual imagery in my day-to-day life too, which reduced my anxiety a lot. Eventually it felt as though the load I was carrying became a lot lighter. I became calmer.

Everything had been clouded and difficult up to that point. I'd had a strong fear that I would never have a baby. But I'd also had a strong fear of falling pregnant and everything going wrong. The hypnotherapy helped me to become clear again about what I wanted. For the first time in ages, I started to enjoy the idea of a little person growing inside me.

Finally pregnant

Because of all the problems I'd had with my pregnancies, I went back to see my obstetrician to make sure that I had all my bases covered. On one particular day I was due to visit him, and my period was late. The longest my cycle had ever stretched out to was 40 days – and it was now more that that. So I did a test that morning, just to be sure. Negative. Again.

So off I went, and the obstetrician wrote out a prescription for me for hormone tablets. I picked them up from the pharmacy straightaway.

But that evening I thought, *I really should have my period by now*. For some reason I felt different. I had a gut feeling that I was pregnant. I thought I should do another test just to be sure.

This time the result was different. Two lines. Two of them!

I brought the test out to the living room and said, 'Bill, look at this.'

'Oh ... okay,' he said, very low key.

It was almost two years since we had lost our third pregnancy. This was amazing news. But we were both in disbelief. Eventually, fear set in. We were scared about the future and fearful we would end up back at the beginning.

The gift

I continued to see my hypnotherapist while I was pregnant. That was when the most powerful session of all took place.

She worked with me on visualising a new little spirit being given to me by the three that had passed before it. During this process, I acknowledged that maybe this pregnancy was going to work. This little guy was ready for us, and we were ready for him. And even more importantly, he had three little guardian angels protecting him every step of the journey. I could see that our baby was going to be just fine! And yes, at this point the tissues couldn't come fast enough.

I also did an exercise which allowed me to choose a path to follow. I could see very clearly a bright, happy, positive path and one that was dark and difficult. I could choose to go down the hard path if I really wanted to … but the choice was obvious. It was finally time for that bright path.

Waiting

The time disappeared so fast during my pregnancy. I was working like a mad woman and often slipped back into denial, despite this beautiful thought that – just maybe – we would be lucky enough to have a baby of our own.

While logic tells you it will be okay, and healthy babies are born each day, we refused to make it real. We were afraid the odds were still against us. Bill probably struggled with it even more than I did. At least I'd had the hypnotherapy, so I could enjoy a quiet excitement about the pregnancy. Bill didn't have that kind of support. He is a sensitive, quiet soul and never makes a fuss. But he really struggled through those three years, and his reaction to the pregnancy was evidence of how hard it had been on him.

It wasn't until I was 25 weeks' pregnant that he finally had enough confidence to read the weekly update from a pregnancy book I had bought.

Every now and again he would put his hand on my belly and talk to the baby. With a mixture of fear and hope, he would say, 'If you can hear me in there, just letting you know that we can't wait to see you.' He often kept it lighthearted, telling the baby, 'I hope you don't get my nose and ears,' and 'You'd better represent our country!'

The nursery reflected where we were really at. It was just an empty bedroom until a few weeks before our baby arrived. The pram was our first purchase. How scary – it seemed way too real.

If it hadn't been for an incredible family, our baby wouldn't have had anything to wear. Even the car seat wasn't bought until after our baby was born. That would have completely jinxed everything! Bill and I were so oblivious to the world of babies that when it came time to bring our beautiful little boy home we had to ask someone to tell us how to lengthen the straps on the baby seat!

Coming home

As soon as I walked through our back door with our new babe in arms, I suddenly remembered a dream I'd had about a year earlier. I had dreamed of a happy little toddler zooming around on our recently laid courtyard. It was a boy with a funny little grin. That dream had given me such hope. But I'd forgotten all about it until that moment. All I could do was quietly sob, with happiness and absolute relief.

How lucky we are to have this precious, precious little miracle. Not a day has gone by that Bill and I haven't looked at each other with pride and sheer delight. How grateful we are to enjoy this beautiful gift each day, and to know that his three guardian angels are never far away.

* Real names were replaced with pseudonyms in this story.

7
Jane's story

HAVE YOU EVER HEARD OF EXTENDED ADOLESCENCE? WELL, I personified it. At age 30 I was travelling around the Caribbean islands, teaching English by day, dancing on the beach at night, as free as a bird. This was after a decade of exploring the world. I was hooked on travel, and having an amazing time. The last words that would have entered my vocabulary were 'biological clock'.

The idea of finding a husband wasn't on my mind either. I'd never met a guy who was the marrying kind, and I was fine with being single. So it's ironic what happened next.

When the days and nights of the Caribbean drew to a close, I returned to my home town. Soon after, I saw my ex-neighbour at a party – a guy called Colin. All that time as neighbours we had been nothing more than friends. He was now living in a big city 1000 kilometres away. It was utterly inconvenient, but we fell in love.

Colin and I spent two years commuting before I moved cities to be with him.

I had always assumed I'd have kids one day, but it had never been at the forefront of my mind. Being with Colin, I started to see it as a possibility for the first time.

It dawned on me that I was now in my thirties, and maybe I didn't have all that much time on my side. But it was a fleeting thought, and I definitely wasn't in any hurry.

A great lifestyle

I married Colin when I was 35 and he was 38. But you wouldn't say that we settled down. We were living in a great apartment overlooking the ocean. We would go out to good restaurants. We often had weekends away. We had great friends, dinner parties, and regularly crewed on yachts. Life was pretty good.

There was also a lot happening on the career front for me. I had moved out of teaching and into marketing. It had taken a long time, and I'd done a masters degree to get there. But finally I had landed this great marketing job. I was working long hours and my job involved lots of socialising. My boss really loved a drink. He often reconvened work meetings at the pub. And we'd often go out for lunch with a client and end up staying all afternoon drinking.

Motherhood wasn't a natural fit with all of this. But I thought it would happen eventually, when the time was right. I assumed I'd have a large degree of control over when that time was.

Although I wasn't ready for motherhood at that point, I began some preparation. I had my rubella shot and I upgraded my health insurance to cover maternity costs.

I also went off the pill. We used other contraception in the meantime. I didn't want to take any chances because I assumed that unprotected sex would lead to pregnancy within a matter of months.

So we were good to go ... but not just yet.

Hubby ready

Colin was initially the one who felt ready. I knew we should probably start soon, since I was 35. But for some reason I felt a strong resistance to it.

To be honest, I still wasn't feeling any hint of a biological clock. And I really wanted to keep my career going. So I found a few excuses to put it off. We had planned a weekend away in a beautiful wine region, so I suggested we wait until after that so I could enjoy all the food and wine without worrying about whether I might be pregnant. Then I thought I should wait until the end of a big product launch that was coming up at work. It would involve travelling around the country, working fourteen-hour days and heading out afterwards for obligatory drinking sessions.

Colin was upset that I kept postponing it. But in my mind I was thinking, *We'll be right!* I didn't think a few extra months would make a difference.

I also wanted to be healthy and stress-free when we started trying. And that would require a reasonably big transition because my work was just so full on.

Am I ready?

After the product launch, I ran out of excuses. And because of my age, I thought we were running out of time. I still didn't feel 100 percent ready, but I knew it was time to get on with it.

I thought we would just do away with the condoms and it would happen. I had no idea about the timing of my cycle. I had no idea when I was ovulating. I never thought I would need to know this stuff!

> As even more time went by, I realised that making a baby wasn't as easy as I'd thought it would be.

Three or four months into it, I thought it was strange that I hadn't become pregnant. So it was only then that I started keeping track of my periods.

As even more time went by, I realised that making a baby wasn't as easy as I'd thought it would be. It became clear that I had quite a long and unpredictable cycle. So I gradually introduced a few 'tricks' which I thought might help us to get pregnant.

Trick number one was the saliva ovulation test. I would lick a microscope slide, and if it formed fern-like patterns I was apparently ovulating. But for some reason it would form fern-like patterns several times throughout the cycle. Not particularly helpful.

So I introduced another trick. I started weeing on sticks – the ones that tell you when you're about to ovulate. There were only four sticks in the pack, which were supposed to be used on consecutive days. In the five or six weeks of my cycle, choosing the right four days was a bit like picking winning Lotto numbers.

I also started to take my temperature every morning and plot the results on a graph. I could see that my temperature did increase at a certain point in the cycle, which is apparently what happens when you ovulate. But every month that point in the cycle would change. So it didn't actually help me predict when I would be ovulating.

All these things were supposed to be helping. But instead, they added to a growing sense of frustration. Although I hadn't initially been in love with the idea of motherhood, I had nevertheless made a decision to get pregnant. So I wanted to do everything I could to make it happen. That's just in my nature – when I set out to do something, I do it properly, and I cover all bases.

Before we had started trying to have a baby, sex had always been a way of feeling close. It had also been free and spontaneous. If we felt like spending the day in bed together, we'd do it. If we got home from a great night out and felt like being together, we would. And if we were feeling tired, it didn't matter if we went for a couple of weeks without having sex. But now it had turned into a routine, scheduled, constant thing. Get the legs in the air and here we go again.

On a physical level, it was exhausting having to do that all the time. And it wore me down emotionally as well.

Information overload

Around this time, a friend lent me a pile of books on the subject of conception. I read them obsessively, thinking, *The answer's in here somewhere. What am I doing wrong?*

Oh, shit! I wasn't supposed to drink at all. I wasn't supposed to have any stress. Apparently I had to wrap myself in cotton wool, eat mung beans and drink filtered water. My husband would have to do the same. Then, maybe, we would have a chance. But because of our ages, it was still only a 'maybe'.

The information started to do my head in. It wasn't surprising that Col told me to get rid of the bloody books! But one good thing did come out of my little research mission – I decided to cut down my alcohol intake.

> I wasn't supposed to have any stress. Apparently I had to wrap myself in cotton wool, eat mung beans and drink filtered water.

Time for help

I was 36 by now. When you're a bit older, instead of waiting twelve months to see a doctor about fertility issues, intervention tends to occur after six months. So off I went to see my gynaecologist.

He began the process by giving me an unsolicited social commentary. 'I see a lot of women who leave it till their late thirties,' he told me. 'They wait for the perfect man. They want it all – the perfect husband and career. But you can't have it all. If you leave it too late, you run the risk of it taking much longer to fall pregnant.'

You can imagine my reaction. I said, 'I can't help the fact that I didn't meet a guy I could marry until this age! That's how my life has panned out.'

To check if everything was okay, I ended up having a laparoscopy. (Basically, that is where they go in with a little camera and check out all your plumbing.) They found that everything was fine. There was a superficial patch of endometriosis, but they were able to clear that up. There was also a slight case of polycystic ovary syndrome. Apparently that would only be a problem if it stopped me from ovulating. For now, at least, it wasn't an issue.

I was used to the idea that if you worked hard enough you always got what you wanted. So this was baffling to me. I was working my way down a checklist, doing all the right things. I was eating healthy food, exercising, cutting down on alcohol, getting checked out by a doctor. I was almost living in a bubble trying to get pregnant!

Having checked off everything on my list, I moved on to Colin. I made him go and have his sperm tested. They discovered that they were mostly swimming in the right direction. But I started to give him a hard time whenever he drank too much. The poor guy! We were eight or nine months into it by now. We would go out to a restaurant and order a bottle of wine. I would have one glass, and Col might finish the rest of the bottle. And I would say, 'What are you doing? We're trying to get pregnant!'

I can see now that I was a complete nightmare. My obsessing was causing a strain on our relationship. We would go for long walks on the weekends and we would discuss – no, *I* would discuss – what we were doing wrong. I would switch into analysis mode. What else could we try that might work? How about we look into Chinese medicine? Why are other people my age falling pregnant on their first try? And how on earth did my friend fall pregnant by accident, when here I am doing everything in my power to make it happen?

Colin would patiently humour me. Of course, he would get frustrated too, at times, that we weren't falling pregnant. But in his mind it was normal for it to take a year or more at our age. He believed there was nothing wrong with us, and a bit of alcohol wasn't going to hurt.

The stakes

As time went on, I started to think, *What if I can't get pregnant?* Now, that was a really scary thought. There was one reason in particular that it scared me: I was adopted.

I've never found my biological parents. It's not a big issue for me – I adore my adoptive parents. But in trying to conceive my own child, some unexpected emotions came up.

If I could have a baby, I knew I would be able to look into another human being's eyes, and for the first time in my life I would be looking at someone who was related to me; my own flesh and blood. What if that never happened? I would never know anyone else in the world who was part of me, biologically.

> If I could have a baby, I knew I would be able to look into another human being's eyes, and for the first time in my life I would be looking at someone who was related to me

These thoughts made me a bit teary occasionally. And they became a driving force for me, making me even more determined to conceive.

But there was another layer of pressure on top of that. My mum was ill with bowel cancer at the time, and she was going through a long bout of depression. So she and Dad were sharing my disappointment month after month, desperately wanting some good news in their lives.

At one stage, during a phone call to Dad, I said, 'Mum would be so happy if I just got pregnant.'

'Jane, it would cure her!' he said, without thinking.

My heart sank. Now I thought I had to try to do this for Mum, as much as for Col and me.

Something's got to give

Even with all of this going on, I was still working hard. I was spending a long time commuting, and during the day I was so busy I didn't even have time to pee.

The whole time I had an underlying feeling of guilt. I thought I shouldn't be working so hard. And even though the social side of work had calmed down a bit, I also thought I shouldn't be drinking as much as I was.

Then fate intervened to change everything.

Colin was given an opportunity to work in my home town. It was a much smaller city and my family, and lots of old friends, were still living there. Colin thought that if were starting a family, it would be fantastic to have all of those people around.

At first I didn't want to leave our amazing life in the big city. And I was reluctant to resign from my job because I had worked so hard to establish that new career. By moving away, we would be closing that fantastic chapter of our lives and committing fully to the next chapter – family life.

We had been trying to conceive for a year, and on a practical level I was committed to it, to the point of obsession. Yet there was another side of me that still hadn't really committed to it.

> Although I wanted to have a family with Colin, the thought of a domestic life in the suburbs with babies wasn't doing it for me.

Although I wanted to have a family with Colin, the thought of a domestic life in the suburbs with babies wasn't doing it for me. I had reached my mid-thirties, and I'd spent fifteen years travelling around, doing my own thing and being really independent. I'd heard stories about what it was like to have kids, and they often made me stop and think: *Do I really want this?*

Your life is over, I would hear. You'll spend all your time at home. You won't sleep at night. Your career will be stuffed.

I tried not to think about these things too much, because if I had let myself go down that track, I might actually have stopped trying.

In the end, we decided to make a permanent move back to my home town. The debate in my head was silenced (or at least hushed). By moving interstate, I was committing fully to the path of conception and motherhood.

That was all good and well – but there was still a huge question mark in relation to our fertility.

In vitro fertilisation

Infertility – or sub-fertility – are such hideous labels. They can start to define you. As we moved cities, it felt like I had this great big sign hanging above my head saying 'INFERTILE'.

As soon as we arrived, I booked in to see someone about IVF. But there was more than a three-month wait to get in to see the doctor. What a blow! I was so desperate for answers, I even started asking the receptionist at the IVF clinic for her advice.

Even though we had to wait, the fact that I made that IVF appointment gave me a psychological edge. I thought, *I've tried everything in my power. Now I'm going to have the medical profession on my side too. We're going to get this done.*

> It was the Christmas period, so I decided not to look for work for a couple of months. My body finally had a chance to de-stress.

I have to admit, it really helped that I wasn't working any more. It was the Christmas period, so I decided not to look for work for a couple of months. My body finally had a chance to de-stress.

Since I wasn't working, I threw all of my energy into house hunting. I looked at properties every single day, and it completely took my focus off getting pregnant. Colin encouraged me to take a day off, but I didn't want to. I was in the zone; loving my new mission.

It was only a matter of weeks before we bought a great new home, just up the road from a groovy café strip. With a new house, my parents in the same city, and so many old friends close by, that life in the 'burbs suddenly didn't seem so dreary.

A bit of spontaneity

I can actually pinpoint the occasion on which we conceived. It's funny to look back on it now, because it was very spontaneous. It felt quite different to all those nights of 'trying'.

We had gone away for the weekend to a beautiful little country town. I can't really explain why, but over breakfast I just sensed something – I knew I was ovulating. I had never had that feeling before.

I happened to make a visit to the bathroom, and I discovered there was lots of the clear stuff. So I returned to the table with a new look in my eye.

'It's now, Col. It's now!' I said.

> Looking after a baby is damned hard work but what an amazing experience! It's a love of the most extraordinary kind.

I'll keep the details between my husband and me. But suffice to say, we rushed out of the café, found a suitable location in the great outdoors, laughed a hell of a lot … and *voilà*!

One of the happiest phone calls I have ever made was to the receptionist at the IVF clinic.

'I don't need you now. I'm pregnant!' I told her.

In fact, I'd become pregnant within a month of making the appointment.

Round two

I'm now 38, and I work from home while looking after my one-year-old boy.

My mum comes over all the time to be with him. After five really tough years her depression has lifted and her cancer is in remission. She is smiling and laughing again and I think her beautiful new grandson has a lot to do with it. When she sees him, she is full of life and her eyes shine. It really has changed her life. And my dad is like a young man again!

Of course, it has changed my life too. It has been a challenge, but I've settled into my role as a working mum. I have to say that conceiving, carrying and giving birth to a child blows away any travel story, study or work achievement. Looking after a baby is damned hard work but what an amazing experience! It's a love of the most extraordinary kind.

Now Colin and I are starting to try for baby number two. I'm much more relaxed about conceiving this time around, because I know we can do it now. And miraculously, my periods have taken on a nice, predictable 30-day cycle! Who would have thought?

Postscript: Within three months of being interviewed for this book, Jane was pregnant again. She reports that, this time, no sticks were weed on, no microscope slides licked, no temperatures taken and no ovulation kits used.

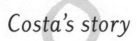

Costa's story

IT'S SUCH A WEIRD THING WHEN YOU LOOK BACK ON IT. YOU FINISH school, play in a band, find work, have some of the best days of your life with lifelong mates of both sexes, get drunk, get stoned, get laid, travel and generally don't give too much thought to what's going on around you. And suddenly you're thirty.

Things start to get serious. Those lifelong mates have hooked up with lifelong mates of their own. Some have dropped off along the way, some naturally, some tragically. And one of those friends you've decided to build a life with.

In your twenties your plans didn't look much past the following weekend. But now here you are with a gold ring and a mortgage. Yes, somehow you've convinced a man in a suit to lend you a ridiculous sum of money.

The next thing you know, some of your friends are starting families. Some better planned than others. And that's how it all begins.

My wife and I don't get caught up in the baby thing straightaway. We want to get everything in place and do it when we feel ready.

That readiness kicks in at about thirtyish. Okay. Let's start a family. Can't be that hard. Bit of fun really. People do it all the time.

Fertility blues

After twelve months of unfruitful though enjoyable 'trying' we're getting anxious. I'm a little concerned and my wife is *more* than a little concerned. We go off to the medical professionals and we get tested.

I'm pretty happy with the sperm count results. They're normal. Phew. My wife has some basic tests, including one which checks the compatibility of my sperm with her cervical mucus. All looks A.O.K. The doctor gives her a drug called clomid to help with fertility and tells us to go away for six months.

Three months roll by. My wife has a gut instinct; something is wrong here. Let's get a second opinion. This time she insists on a more thorough examination. She books in for a laparoscopy. It shows she has severe endometriosis and both her tubes are blocked. We wouldn't have had a hope in hell if this had gone undetected. My wife's energy deflates like a balloon with a slow leak. She has gone from being told 'There is no problem here' to 'We *might* be able to help you get pregnant.'

Time to embark on some assisted reproduction options. But we're steadfastly keeping it to ourselves. The last thing we need is everyone asking whether we've been successful with our last treatment or not.

However, as much as you try to keep it to yourself, inevitably questions are asked and people find out. I swear I'll never ask anyone: 'When are you going to start a family?' It's such a personal question. I'm sure we've all asked it at one time or another, but I know I never will again. The feelings that question can conjure are many and varied, but mostly one of two: you want to choke the living shit out of whoever asked you, or sit in a corner and have a good cry.

In a lot of ways, we men have it relatively easy when the downstairs action goes a bit awry. We may have to change some of our recreational activities that aren't so good for the sperm count, like a good binge on Saturday night. And we may even have to go from underpants to boxer shorts – apparently tight, white ball huggers keep your boys too warm – but it's our partners who have to put in most of the effort, especially when you start heading down the medical road.

Our first attempt is a procedure called GIFT (gamete intra-fallopian transfer). This is where eggs are removed from the ovary and placed with sperm in the fallopian tube, where it's hoped they will fertilise naturally, as opposed to being put together in a dish beforehand. The doctor advises us to put two eggs in for our first go.

We do a pregnancy test two weeks later.

'Positive!'

'Really?'

'Yes, really.'

That's our first look at a positive pregnancy test after so many negative ones in the year we attempted to conceive naturally. To say we're excited and happy is an understatement. This time it has actually worked.

We try to keep it to ourselves and for the most part do. Big smiles, but still a bit nervous. Then we're off for the scan. Bad news. Blighted ovum. Both of them. Seems that we're learning all the time. A blighted ovum is where the foetus has died at a very early stage and there is no heartbeat. We had a 100 percent success rate with the fertilisation of the two eggs, but neither of them lasted.

From the top of the world back down to earth. Once again you tell yourself to look on the bright side, at least the eggs fertilised. What happens next? A curette. What's that? They have to scrape out the uterus to clean it out. An abortion of sorts. Out of all the ups and downs, this one really knocks us around. We thought we'd got there, only to have the rug pulled from under us.

We're told to go home and come back first thing in the morning for the curette. That night my wife is in excruciating pain but she keeps thinking she only has to get through the night. It will all be over in the morning.

The next day, we're off to the hospital and reality sets in. The doctor tells her the pain has been caused by a miscarriage and it will settle down soon.

My wife stays in hospital that night and I do what a lot of guys possibly do – go to a party and have a few drinks. I'm not in much of a party mood but I go along anyway. It's a going away party for a good mate who I'm not likely to see for many years. And what's the point of going home and drinking alone?

About a week later I'm at work. I usually am when all the big things happen. The house floods, washing machine blows up, switchboard catches fire. Yep, at work every time. And sometimes not even in the same city. I have a late night national radio program to host, can't let the metalheads (my listeners) down. It's not like I can walk into the boss and say: 'Gotta go.'

I receive a phone call from my sister-in-law while I'm on-air. My wife is in terrible pain and on her way to the hospital.

When they arrive, she's given something for the pain which only just takes the edge off it. They do a scan. Can't find anything wrong. The doctors have her history so they know exactly what they're looking for but still can't work it out. Curette went without a hitch. Are you constipated? No. Better get the apparatus out just in case. A good bowel clean out and still the pain persists.

Then she is told, 'Looks like you need your appendix out.' Back into surgery. But it turns out the appendix is okay. So what's the problem? An ectopic pregnancy. That's the development of a fertilised egg in a fallopian tube. Back when the two eggs were implanted, one of them split in two – both parts were fertilised and found their way to the uterus. The other egg was also fertilised, but ended up lodging in the tube. We didn't know about that until now. The doctors say it's one of the worst pains you can experience.

IVF time

After a while we're on to in vitro fertilisation – in other words, putting the sperm and egg together in a dish.

My wife gets up at 5 a.m. to be at the clinic by 6 a.m. to get hormone injections five days a week, and maybe a bit of a look around by the gloved doctor before heading off to work.

For the man, bringing your half of the IVF equation to the lab is a fairly simple process. At our particular clinic I'm advised not to do it in the comfort of my own environment. Fresh is best and, after all, there is a room with a comfy chair, whale music if you choose (I don't), a selection of rather explicit magazines and most importantly, a door that locks from the inside.

Time is always the enemy in a situation like this. You ring the bell to alert the scientist in the lab that you need your specimen jar. Obviously you don't want to ring that bell again too soon to give him the said specimen. But you have been saving this up for a while and those mags do have an interesting effect. Did I say time is your enemy? Gravity isn't exactly your best mate either ...

> Going to the local pharmacy to get a sharps kit for needle disposal is, however, a little confronting.

When it's done and bottled you ring the bell again and you're not sure who you want to answer the door. But in the end it's just a job, you've done yours, now it's their turn to do theirs, which will hopefully mean putting together some viable embryos. Not the conventional way to get this particular job done but you come to realise at this point that the rule book has been thrown out the window and you're really just a cog in a scientific wheel with about a 20 percent chance of success.

After a while we decide it would be best for me to give my wife the needles to avoid at least some of the 5 a.m. starts. To start with, it's a strange experience pinching up a bit of fat on her tummy and injecting it. But after a while I start to enjoy playing nurse.

Going to the local pharmacy to get a sharps kit for needle disposal is, however, a little confronting. People tend to give you a look which says 'another junkie', but I never make a point of explaining myself. What business is it of theirs anyway?

My needling skills don't get us all the way though. There is one needle she needs on the day before the embryo transfers that I'm not allowed to give. She is asked to come to the clinic at the convenient hour of 2 a.m. for this one. Like I said, the boys do get off rather easily.

Even as a male, the fertility stuff consumes your thoughts a fair bit when you're going through IVF. My emotions take me by surprise when I see a father and his child holding hands walking down the street or playing at the park and I wonder whether I'll ever have that experience. Ever feel that love.

'We had sex once and I was pregnant.' Boy do those words rattle around in your head when you've been heading to the IVF clinic for over a year and the medical bills are mounting.

My wife is quite desperate about the whole thing. It's my job to add a bit of levity and stay positive. Even though you can feel pretty redundant medically, the man comes into his own on this emotional battle line. When faced with another negative cycle, sometimes there is just nothing left to do or say. The best thing you can be is a shoulder, a punching bag or a yelling post. But best to just be there.

Changes

After about 18 months and multiple procedures, my enthusiasm is really starting to wane but best not mention it. I'm actually starting to think that our lot in life is to remain childless, buy a dog and go overseas every couple of years. Sounds pretty attractive. But something, I'm not sure what, drives me to keep going. I honestly think that drive is more prevalent in the female of the species. Maybe that's why I keep going. I really couldn't bear to tell my wife that I've had enough.

We press on with the IVF. But finally we come to the realisation that something has to give and it's our lifestyle. We can't keep going on like this if we're going to succeed in starting a family.

We both have pretty demanding jobs with long hours. My long hours are generally taken up going to see bands and networking with industry people, so it's hardly work. My wife's job is constant. She's still in the office at 10 p.m. most nights. We decide she should quit her job and concentrate on baby making.

Emotionally there is a lot going on for her as well. Neither of her parents is well. And did I mention our goldfish has just died?

Let's just relax and take it easy. We'll survive on one wage.

When she does finally finish work, I feel like I'm living with a different person. A far more contented individual.

Another treatment clicks past. I travel across the country for work and my wife comes to join me for a holiday when my work obligations are over. We catch up with friends, visit wilderness reserves and do touristy things. The four-wheel-drive tracks and corrugations in the dirt roads probably don't do our cause much good but we have one of the best holidays ever. We both find ourselves forgetting about the constant grind of work, IVF and everything else that's been going on at home. I even do a tandem parachute jump. When I land on the beach my wife runs up to me and says, 'Princess Diana has just been killed in a car crash.'

'I don't give a shit. I just jumped out of a plane!'

Clearly, I'm not Mr Popular with the English backpackers who happen to be within earshot.

I get back home and my boss calls me to ask if I want to go to a major city to act in a management position for six months. Don't have to think about that one for too long. We both love our home town, but it's getting us down. It feels like family pressures and our hectic schedules are working against us. Normally we would cope okay with these things, but with the added pressure of IVF, things are starting to close in around us. Let's go. Let's see what the big city is like.

The plan is for me to live in an apartment for three weeks while I look for something more permanent. Then my wife will move down. She can have one more treatment before moving, and that will leave us with two frozen embryos to go.

On my first weekend I'm walking around the city checking out the sights. My wife is scheduled to have some embryos implanted some time this morning. By this stage we're pretty blasé about the whole thing because we've been through it so many times.

We've only ever put in two embryos at a time. For quite a while the doctor has been suggesting that the odds are better if you put three back in. I've been steadfastly against it. One of my friends has just had identical twin boys and that was plenty to deal with. I can't contemplate having triplets. But my wife has been thinking about it seriously for the last couple of cycles, and I've finally relented. Let's face it, neither of us is getting any younger.

I'm walking along, sightseeing, when my phone rings. It's my mother-in-law. I know straightaway something is amiss.

'Everything is okay,' she says.

'What do you mean everything is okay?'

'They had a bit of a problem. She's had a reaction to the anaesthetic. You'd better give the doctor a call.'

I take down the number. I hang up the phone and my knees buckle under me. I don't quite kiss the cement but I come close. I find a quiet laneway, have a little blub and call the doctor. He tells me what happened – an anaphylactic shock, which is an extreme reaction to one of the drugs the anaesthetist gave her. Oddly, the same cocktail of drugs she has had every other time.

'Should I come back?' I ask.

'Not much point. She's out of danger now but it was touch and go for a while. If you're going to have an anaphylactic shock, the operating table is a good place to have it. We put the embryos in but I don't think there'll be much chance this time.'

I finally speak to my wife. We're both completely spun out and vow that this is our last go. It's not worth losing your life over.

To be focused on this one outcome, and then to have it nearly take your wife's life away, is a rude shock. I don't want to have anything to do with IVF. For me it's over. The risks have outweighed the benefits. I want kids but I want my wife more.

It's not as cut and dried for my wife. She knows we still have two frozen embryos. In the back of her mind she thinks she'll probably use them. There is that single-minded determination again.

We don't think for a minute that the implantation could possibly have worked. We put it out of our minds. My wife more or less packs up the house by herself and joins me in our new home, which happens to be a shoebox. At least it's a shoebox located near the beach. We settle into our new surroundings. Life is pretty fine.

We both have a new sense of freedom – no-one around to tell us what we should do or where we should go. We just jump in the car and drive. Neither of us has ever lived in a different city from our families. For the first time in our lives, our only real responsibility is to ourselves and our cat, Barney.

> I don't want to have anything to do with IVF. For me it's over. The risks have outweighed the benefits. I want kids but I want my wife more.

Pregnant?

About three weeks after the implantation, my wife realises that she hasn't even bothered to do a pregnancy test. She decides to do one but she won't look at it – can't bear to see another negative result. So I look.

'Is it supposed to be a plus sign?' I ask.

'Yeah.'

'Well, it's positive.'

'It's not!'

'It is!'

Neither of us can believe our eyes. Maybe this time, against the odds, we've jagged it!

Friday morning. Better go and do some shopping, have to work tonight. I draw the short straw and leave my wife at home. She starts bleeding. She has no idea where the nearest hospital is. Calls my phone and hears it ring in the bedroom. *Damn, he left it here.* She calls a cab that drops her off at the nearest medical centre. It's closed. She jumps in another one and goes to a different medical centre. Sees a doctor. 'You had better go and have a scan at a diagnostic centre in the next suburb,' he says.

I get home, see her note and jump back in the car. Finally find her trying to hail a cab. 'What's going on?' She fills me in and we bumble our way to the diagnostic centre. We find a car park, only to realise that the numbers on this particular road go sequentially from one end to the other. So 256 isn't across the road from 257 – it's about 3 kilometres in the other direction. Back in the car, we find the right place and this time I can't find a car park, so I just drop off my wife and go in search of one.

I find my way back to the centre. By the way, to have one of these scans it's best to have a full bladder, so my wife has drunk three litres of water in about half an hour. Because of our situation she jumps the queue and she's in there before I make it inside.

It seems to take forever and the poor girl next to me who has drunk her requisite three litres has just been gazumped by us. She's in dire need to be rid of some of that water but can't just yet.

Better call the boss, the metalheads will have to miss out tonight. I'm wondering what else can be thrown at us. Haven't we passed the test yet? Surely having children will be a doddle after all this.

Twenty minutes later my wife finally walks out with a massive smile on her face and holds up three fingers. Let's see, three o'clock, three hundred dollars, three babies. Nah, couldn't be. She promptly walks into another room and leaves me sitting there wondering. Meanwhile bladder girl finally gets the call and can barely walk to the room for her scan.

Out comes my wife and I say 'Three what?'

'Three heartbeats.'

'Really?'

'Really.'

Still that huge smile on her face.

I feel a mixture of elation with a dash of euphoria and a good dose of terror. I'm going to be a father. Of three. Holy shit! How are we ever going to cope with triplets?

I still don't go to work that night. We just sit at home with our takeaway. We keep looking at each other and saying, 'Three?' And, 'Oh my God, triplets!'

I watch my wife grow. And grow she does. She has another bleed and, yes, I am away in another city at the time. She finds her own way to the hospital.

Our time in the big city comes to an end and we say our goodbyes. Back at home, my wife is ordered to have bed rest for a good portion of the pregnancy. She gets so big that I have to help her out of bed at night to go to the toilet.

We're 31 weeks in. Our obstetrician has said that 35 would be a good number. By this stage my wife is having weekly scans and this one presents a bit of a problem. Triplet three (later to become known as Holly) is in distress. There is a problem with her umbilical cord.

Doctor says, 'This is going to happen sooner rather than later.'

'What's sooner rather than later?'

'How soon can you get home, pack and get back here?'

'An hour.'

'See you then.'

A scan that afternoon confirms that the babies will be born the following day. It will be a caesarean, as it's a bit iffy doing it naturally when there are three of them.

My wife spends the night in hospital and I go back to work in a daze. It's not one of my better shows. I go home and contemplate what the rest of my life is going to be like. Nothing like the first 34 years I'm sure.

Surreal is the best way of describing how I feel when I wake on Saturday, 9 May, knowing that in a couple of hours I'll be a father of three. I drive to the hospital and meet my wife and the doctor. She gets prepped and the doctor and I scrub up. I know he means business when he puts on a pair of white gum boots.

There are probably ten people in the theatre. A team for each of the kids, the doctor, the registrar, my wife and me. I'm sitting next to my wife. Neither of us can see anything behind a sheet they erect between us and the operation. From behind the sheet, the doctor holds up a baby and says: 'It's a girl!' About a minute later: 'It's a boy!'

'I can't see anything,' I say.

'Stand up,' he tells me.

I stand up and see the most amazing sight of all time. The doctor pulls a sac from my wife's now semi-deflated stomach, holds it in his left palm, taps it with his scalpel, fluid goes everywhere and there is Holly in the palm of his hand. 'It's a girl!'

They're all pretty healthy but it's off to intensive care to be put in humidicribs. Rebecca and Josh are 1.6 kilograms (3 lb, 9 oz) and Holly is 1.2 kilograms (2 lb, 11 oz). They're all tiny. Holly, the smallest, is in an open cot under lights and bubble wrap to keep her warm. We were supposed to have a look around intensive care before we had the kids so it wouldn't freak us out, but I didn't make it. Yep, it's a pretty freaky place. Lots of machines that go bing and dedicated nurses and doctors, and happy/sad parents.

I meet the doctor in my wife's room a couple of hours later and you couldn't whack the smile off my face with a baseball bat. He says, 'That all went pretty well but the next 24 hours will be crucial.'

That almost wipes the smile off.

Even so, my wife and I look at each other and think, *We've done it. We actually pulled it off.* They're tiny but we think they're going to be okay.

They stay in hospital for about six weeks while they get fatter and we get things organised at home. We purposely haven't bought anything or made up a nursery because the last thing we wanted was to have everything set up for three babies and only bring one or two home, which was a real possibility.

Being a dad

The first three months are a complete blur of bottles, nappies, sterilisers, vomit (mostly Josh's) and other malodorous objects.

Actually the first two years become a blur.

I never realised that having a child brings with it a whole new kind of love. It feels unconditional and everlasting but it's also kind of scary at the same time. I tell my dad that I'm worrying about the triplets a lot. He says to me, 'Get used to it, son.' And then I think about all the times I came home at ridiculous hours in the morning in various states of sobriety. What must have been going through his head? Got all that to look forward to yet.

They're nine years old now and they're asleep above me as I tap away at the keyboard. Hang on, footsteps; better go and check. All good. Yes, Dad was right. You never stop worrying.

They're well-behaved, polite and courteous children when they're out but when they're home they can sometimes be right little monsters. We have been blessed though, so far we've had few medical problems. They're a bit skinnier than most but they had a skinny start.

Life's still a bit of a blur but we know that we're only going to get one go at this so we're trying to make the most of every day. Before we know it they'll fly the coop and it'll be back to just the two of us again.

Should be a good ride.

Endnote: The practice of implanting more than one embryo is no longer commonplace. In many jurisdictions it is now forbidden by laws and regulations.

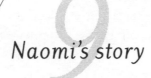

Naomi's story

IT HAD BEEN a BEAUTIFUL LUNCH OF SHELLFISH AND WINE. BUT now I had a terrible stomachache.

'I think I'd better go down to the hospital,' I told my husband, Filip*.

We fronted up to the emergency department and a doctor ran a few tests on me.

'You're not sick,' he concluded. 'You're pregnant.'

'Oh, my God! I have to ring my mum!' I said. After eight and a half years of trying to fall pregnant, they were the first words that came out of my mouth.

We were ridiculously happy, and more than a little shocked. We went through all of the numbers in our phones and rang just about every person to tell them the news.

A long time coming

I knew early on that all was not well 'down south'. Benign cancer cells were removed from my cervix when I was nineteen. I'd also had endometriosis (where the tissue that lines the womb grows beyond the uterus). Cysts were removed from my tubes and ovaries. Because of that physical damage, I always had this thought at the back of my mind: *Maybe I won't be able to have kids.* The idea really knocked my self-confidence around.

Self-confidence had always been an issue for me. I grew up in the country when times were tough. My dad drank a lot. To the outside world, he was a party man. Charming – and funny as hell. It wasn't unusual to come home and find an entire football team standing around having a drink with him. Around the family, it was a different story. A lot of sitting around, quiet and depressed. He was wrapped up in his own world, and didn't always give me the attention I wanted. I used to wish he would notice me; be proud of me.

I was always trying to prove myself. As a kid I pushed myself really hard in swimming and athletics. I became quite competitive. Hard work and achievement meant something. Then, as an adult, my career became important to me.

I never thought I would find someone who would love me enough to marry me. That confidence problem again. But a man called Filip came along and proved me wrong on that front. I was living overseas when we met. One Sunday night I was supposed to go to a friend's party, but I couldn't make it. I turned up on Monday morning to apologise and Filip was still there from the night before. We ended up hanging out for the next three weeks. We drove around the countryside together, and he showed me where he'd gone to school and grown up.

I had to fly home because my dad was ill. Filip and I decided to keep our relationship going. We spoke on the phone a lot, and he sent me a love letter nearly every day.

Dad was in denial about his illness – which turned out to be lung cancer – so there wasn't much for me to do except spend time with him. We didn't have any deep and meaningful conversations, but we managed to grow closer than we had ever been. He accompanied me to the post office a lot when I picked up letters and packages from Filip. He was quite amused by it all.

After a year or so, Filip rang my father to ask if he could marry me. Dad agreed, and when he hung up the phone he joked, 'I hope he doesn't change his mind.'

Filip migrated, and we were married soon after in a secret ceremony with just a few relatives present.

Because we got married so quickly, I suppose there were always a few doubts, mainly on a subconscious level, about how much Filip loved me. The problems I'd had with my reproductive organs played on my mind occasionally. I wondered: *If I can never give this man a child, will he still want to be with me?*

In time we threw a proper wedding reception. Everything was pink, from the flowers to the champagne.

Filip's parents came from overseas to live with us for a year. We all bundled into a two-bedroom house together. I got along well with my father-in-law. We would often sit on the front verandah together chatting about life. My mother-in-law never joined us. She would sit inside watching television or reading.

I had always imagined that if I got married I would be welcomed with open arms into my husband's family. Instead, I felt rejected by my mother-in-law. I assumed she didn't approve of her son's new wife. She'd had nine children, and I probably looked like a career-driven woman who had no desire to make babies or play housekeeper. I wanted to prove myself to her. I thought maybe that would happen when I had children.

When I was about 26, we decided to start trying for a baby. But we were very relaxed about it. Our mindset was: 'If it happens, it happens'. We didn't try to work out when we should have sex. We just played around and waited to see what would happen. On the surface, we are both easy-going people, so it seemed natural for us to take a relaxed approach. But deep down, I was trying to protect myself. I didn't want to take it too seriously. Because what if I gave it my best shot ... and I failed? I'd been able to achieve everything else in my life that I'd ever set out to do. The possibility of failing frightened me.

My way of coping with a problem is typically to forget about it. Quite deliberately, I didn't think about conception or babies much in those early years when we were trying to conceive. Filip and I were having a lot of fun, going to parties, immersing ourselves in our jobs.

I was working long hours in the TV and film industry. Everything had to be done pronto. 'We need lights now.' 'Get the catering sorted.' 'Check the weather for tomorrow's shoot.' The only time I relaxed was in my sleep.

The conception issue only really smacked me in the face when people I knew started having babies. *I'm the only one having trouble conceiving*, I thought.

My insecurities would pop up when colleagues and friends asked: 'When are you and Filip going to have a baby?'

My standard line was: 'I'm not ready.'

My nan regularly called me and asked when I would be having kids. I'd tell her, 'Nannie, you're not allowed to ask me that. It's like asking when Filip and I are having sex.' That didn't stop her from enquiring. I became skilled at talking so fast, she couldn't get any questions in. And I learnt to pass the phone quickly on to Filip.

By this stage my dad had become quite ill. Although we still weren't trying all that hard, I hoped I would fall pregnant while he was still alive. I thought a grandchild would give him a reason to live. And I suppose I wanted to have a baby so that he would be proud of me.

After a couple of years of trying, I thought Filip and I should check things out from a medical point of view. Filip was tested first – but his sperm were all good (much to his delight).

Then it was my turn to be tested. My examinations revealed severe endometriosis. Aaaagh! Another kick in the guts. *It's all my fault.*

I needed three bouts of laser surgery to remove the endometriosis, with six months between each surgery.

Dad continued to decline, so Filip and I drove to the country every other weekend to spend time with him. He was tired. But I would take him for short outings, especially to his favourite restaurant.

Mum told me that he was reflecting a lot on his life. He was feeling a lot of remorse about the kind of father he had been. *Maybe this is all going to work out*, I told myself. *His cancer will go into remission and we'll start afresh. I'll be able to connect with my dad in a whole new way.*

Dad's health went up and down for a period of time, and so did mine. Driving back from the country one Sunday, I had to get Filip to pull over. The pain from my endometriosis was so strong I had to lie on the side of the road in the foetal position.

Eventually my dad passed away. I was so upset that he never lived to see his own grandchild. But I didn't do a lot of grieving. Not in the 'God, I miss him' kind of way. That would come later. I grieved more about the father I wished I'd had.

> Now removed from big parties and long work hours, I wanted to bring a new life into the world. It was time to stop flapping around and take this seriously.

Sea change

After nearly five years of trying to conceive, Filip was offered a job in a small coastal town. I jumped at the chance to escape the question-and-answer set. And I had been working so hard career-wise, I was ready to chill out.

I started my own business and worked from home, at a much slower pace. Up until now my life had been dominated by work. Now I had time to have a cup of tea; to enjoy my own company. I didn't realise how hard I'd been on myself until I stopped.

With all the extra thinking time, I started to work out how I really felt about having children. Although I had wanted to have a baby when Dad was alive, there had always been part of me that wasn't entirely committed to becoming a mother. I hadn't decided on a heartfelt level that I was ready.

When it dawned on me that we had been trying for five years, a sense of urgency kicked in. *Where did all that time go?* I wondered.

Now removed from big parties and long work hours, I wanted to bring a new life into the world. It was time to stop flapping around and take this seriously.

We started to have more frequent sex.

Quite quickly, I went from being ambivalent about motherhood to being fixated on the idea. I started to feel insanely clucky. I remember walking down the street and seeing mothers with their babies. Suddenly I would feel my heart beating inside me. The anxiety would overcome my whole body. I'd have to stop and take a few deep breaths until the feeling passed.

I started to worry about my physical problems a lot more. *What did I do to bring this on? Why am I being punished?*

I still had that niggling fear that Filip wouldn't love me if I couldn't have a baby. One day at the beach I told him, 'If you want to leave me so you have the chance to become a father with someone else, then you can leave.' I said it in a tongue-in-cheek way, but I was actually serious.

'That's absurd!' he told me. 'You're the one I love. I want to be with you no matter what.' And that was that.

I realised Filip would be completely accepting if we couldn't have children. I was the most important thing to him. He really did love me.

I had a lot more confidence after that conversation. For some reason it enabled me to commit even more wholeheartedly to the idea of having children with Filip.

Our new work schedules gave us a lot more time together. In our new coastal home, Filip and I got to know each other better. We spent lots of time gardening, going to the beach and eating out. We poured love onto our cats, Tiger and Bobby, and our border collie, Joey. I often cradled the cats in my arms as though they were babies. They shared our bed with us, too. We promised ourselves that if we ended up having children, we would buy a king-size bed so that we could all snuggle together in the mornings.

After we had been living on the coast for a while, I went to have a pap smear. My doctor discovered that I had a retroverted uterus. 'How do you get one of these things?' I joked. I felt abnormal.

But I wasn't as devastated as I had been when I found out about the endometriosis. It was more a case of: 'Here we go again. Let's do what we can to deal with it.' I found out a bit more about retroverted uteruses on the Internet. I read somewhere that it might help me to conceive if I stuck my legs in the air after sex. That became part of the routine for us. A part that made us both laugh. (Little did I know, about 20 percent of women have a retroverted uterus, and it's unrelated to infertility. Turns out the 'legs in the air' thing is a bit of an old wives' tale.)

A new attitude

After a couple of years of feeling distraught that I couldn't conceive, things slowly started to change.

I had always worried about what everyone else thought. If I couldn't have a baby, I thought I would have failed in their eyes. But gradually I stopped punishing myself with those thoughts. It probably helped that I was in a new place, spending time with people who didn't know my background. Fewer questions. Less pressure.

It also helped that my business started to do really well. So my self-confidence increased.

For over a decade, I had been so disappointed with my body. Now our new lifestyle was conducive to good health. I was relaxing more and eating healthier foods. I was doing a lot of nurturing physical activities like walking the dog and sailing. I even found myself visualising my body being really healthy.

I had been so focused on my fear that it wouldn't work out – that we wouldn't have kids. But in time I allowed myself to imagine how much fun it would be to have them.

I could see myself pushing a pram around, meeting friends for coffee. I wondered what our baby would look like; what sort of personality she or he would have.

I relaxed into it. I thought, *This is going to be great.* I stopped worrying about my age, because I realised that everything was going to work out okay, whether I had a child or not. And I really got on with life. I threw myself into my work and socialising.

It was probably another year before I found myself in that emergency department with a tummy ache, and the best news that Filip and I had ever received.

We went on to have a baby boy called Marcus. Even as a newborn, you would have to say he was charming.

I fulfilled that daydream I'd had – pushing a pram around and going out for café lattes. But I got bored with that after a few weeks. I could see that my natural instinct was to be a working mum. I hired a nanny three days a week and returned to my usual rushing around, between a new job and my new home life.

With Marcus in the world, I began to wish that Dad was around. I found myself grieving for his death in a new way. If he had been here to meet his grandson, that would have been the beginning of a new relationship between us. Children are amazing catalysts for bringing people together. Maybe Dad and I would have made our peace because of this child. I suddenly wished I had said all sorts of things to him. If only I had sat him down and talked about my childhood. If only I had let him know who I really was – and found out what was really going on for him.

A lot of the love I had for my dad came back at that time, and I really missed him. I even remembered what a great father he had been in my younger years. My fondest memory was sitting with him in a cubby house that he had built for me.

A daughter?

I loved raising a son, but I wanted to experience a relationship with a daughter as well. Being from a huge family himself, Filip was definitely up for more children.

From the time Marcus was born, we didn't bother about contraception. But the idea of going at it like rabbits was foreign to us. We went along with the same easygoing approach we'd had the first time around. Let it happen when it happens.

However, there was a new motivation underlying our relaxed approach this time around. I didn't actually feel ready for another child straightaway. Ideally I would have waited until Marcus was three or four. I wanted to give him a lot of my time before bringing a newborn into the picture.

Another reason we were happy to take our time was that our finances were tighter than they had been in the past.

When Marcus was about three, we travelled overseas to see Filip's family. While I was there, I felt so ill, and unbelievably emotional. I spent one night in bed crying for hours. I was going to the toilet constantly, and throwing up. I went to the doctor to find out what was going on, and he got me to do a pregnancy test.

I stared at the result, repeating in my own head the news the doctor had just given me. *I'm pregnant.*

I raced back to our hotel and told Filip, 'I know why I've been so emotional!'

> I had started to plan my life around this unborn child, and I felt such a loss when those plans were taken away from me.

Back at home, I went in for a check-up and my first ultrasound. Lying on the examination table, I heard the most unexpected words coming from the doctor's mouth. 'The foetus hasn't developed,' he said. It was a blighted ovum. A tiny foetus with no heartbeat. The worst thing was that I hadn't brought Filip along for that appointment. I felt so alone when I walked out of that room.

I had started to plan my life around this unborn child, and I felt such a loss when those plans were taken away from me.

A lot of my friends were having babies at that time, and I really wanted to be a part of that. *What if I don't get pregnant?* I wondered.

What am I going to do with my time while my friends are all doing baby things?

I knew I was ready for another child and, from that moment on, I took conception seriously.

I would look at Marcus and feel a strong desire to bring a brother or sister into his life. I remembered all the fun times I'd had with my brother growing up. I even looked back fondly on the thousands of times he dobbed on me.

At age 37, I went back to see my obstetrician to find out if anything was wrong.

An examination revealed that one of my tubes was completely flat. It would be hard, perhaps impossible, for me to conceive naturally. Yet again my self-esteem copped a battering.

From what I was told, I believed in vitro fertilisation was my only hope.

I started injecting the hormones and doing what was required. My emotions were all over the place and I cried all the time. I was so frightened of the future. *If this doesn't work, I'm stuffed.*

My anxiety was heightened by the fact that this was an expensive process, and we planned to attempt only a few rounds. There was so much riding on each procedure.

It was a tense time between Filip and me. I was annoyed that he was drinking more than I thought he needed to. It felt like the issues from my past were leaking into my life again, as I recalled how much my dad used to drink.

At times I felt like I was doing it all alone. But that wasn't always Filip's fault. Instead of asking for help, I used to bait him to try to prove a point.

'Do you want a lift?' he asked me once when I was about to leave for an appointment.

'No, I'll be okay.'

'Come on, let me give you a lift.'

'No. It's no big deal. Stay and have a sleep. I'll catch a taxi.'

'Okay then.'

I ended up blubbering in the doctor's room that day because I wished Filip was there with me.

Although I had those occasional breakdowns, for the most part I didn't want anyone to see how upset I was. I was able to snap into positive mode and look like I was having a great time. I befriended the admin staff at my specialist's office. I brought them morning tea and always joked around with them. I had a fantastic rapport with my specialist too. I don't know how I would have got through without that lightheartedness, but it was definitely a mask I was wearing.

When my first IVF cycle didn't work out, I felt really lost. But I was somewhat distracted because I was moving into a new job. It was great to have some new scenery. New energy. New people. And my pay went up, taking a lot of the financial worries off my mind.

I often had to leave work for IVF appointments. So eventually I told a few work mates what I was going through. They were really supportive. But I played the comedian with them too – making light of everything that was happening.

My second IVF attempt didn't work either. I felt bitter and disillusioned. I cried in the toilets at work, and anywhere else I could snatch a private moment.

Before my third round of IVF, my mum got on the phone to Filip and told him he needed to support me more. 'She can't do this on her own,' Mum told him.

'Well you wouldn't know it. She always acts so brave,' Filip said.

That phone call gave him a jolt. Until then, he hadn't understood just how intense the IVF process was. I'd never really explained it to him.

Filip came to all of my appointments from then on. He had been wanting to do that all along; he'd just assumed I didn't need him. It felt a lot more real having Filip there. *We're both doing this. It's not just me.*

During the third implantation, my specialist said to me, 'This one is a good one. I can tell.'

Of course, he was only saying that. But I had so much faith in this guy. I hung on to those words, and I genuinely believed in myself for the first time in ages. *I can do this*, I thought. I felt a renewed energy.

I made a decision that I was going to keep doing IVF until I fell pregnant. *Hang the cost. I'll do whatever it takes.*

Sitting at work a couple of weeks later, I received a call from my specialist.

'You'd better come in and see me,' he said.

'What's wrong now?' I joked.

'You're having a baby.'

I called Filip straightaway.

'I had a feeling it was going to work this time,' he told me.

After that phone call, I emailed everyone in my office to share the news.

I loved being pregnant again. I loved the sense that this baby was always with me, moving around. It felt like having a butterfly in my tummy.

In the moment my second baby was born, just before it was handed to me, I said, 'What am I going to call him?'

'It's a girl,' my obstetrician corrected me.

I had always dreamed of calling a baby girl 'Ruby', after my dad's mother. And here she was.

Family of four

Now I realise that the long period of time it took to have Marcus was a gift from God. I had a bit of living to do before I could be a mum. I had to get to know Filip better. And I had to have some fun before settling down.

When it eventually happened, boy was I ready.

When I look back on my time in IVF, it wasn't the procedures that I found difficult. For me, the hardest thing was believing in myself. It's amazing what a difference your specialist can make with just a few reassuring words. And I need to give Filip some credit too! His support during that final round of IVF helped me drop a lot of the anxiety I'd had in previous rounds.

I get along with my mother-in-law better these days too. It's important to me that she's a big part of my children's lives. I've come to see that a lot of our early differences came down to cultural misunderstandings. I was so busy looking for her acceptance I overlooked that rather obvious fact.

If my dad was alive, he would be really proud of the person I have become. He would see I'm a loyal person. Capable. Successful in my career. And a great mum.

* Real names were replaced with pseudonyms in this story.

Anna's story

I ALWAYS WANTED TO BE A MOTHER, AND A GOOD MOTHER. I HAD A very happy childhood myself, so it seemed like a very normal thing to want out of life.

For the first six months that my husband and I were trying to conceive, it was an exciting time. But it didn't take long for the emotional highs and lows to become quite acute. Every time I would get my period, I would go into a hole for 24 hours, feeling like the world was against me and that I was pretty much a failure. Then I would pick myself up, just to get knocked down all over again.

At 33, I was used to having a career. I had always felt in control. So with each month that passed I found it harder to reconcile the fact that I had no control over conception.

I've read enough to know how this works. Both of us are healthy. We're well prepared. I should be able to control this, I thought.

In truth, I don't think I understood the subtleties of the process. I assumed that if we just had sex around the right time, we would fall pregnant. The problem was guessing when the 'right time' was. My periods were always different lengths, and a saliva ovulation kit didn't give me any answers. So after about eight months, my GP suggested recording my temperature. With that came a race to the thermometer every morning. I really believe that was more destructive than helpful. I had hoped that a pattern would emerge with the temperatures I was recording, but it never did.

What's wrong with me, I wondered. *Am I too old?* I hadn't even thought about my age before now, but I'd recently read a few alarming statistics, and my GP had also said, 'You can't really afford to hang around too long at your age …'

In a bit of a panic, I thought, *Why didn't we start this process earlier?* My husband and I had been together for six years before we began trying to conceive. *If you had married me earlier, none of this would have happened*, I reasoned. Of course, that wasn't really correct – it was just one of many thoughts that came out of my frustration and distress.

Although I wondered whether something was wrong, I never considered the possibility that we wouldn't have children. That just wasn't an option.

I wasn't working at that time, so my main focus was on having a baby. I knew that it shouldn't be my priority. But the more I told myself that, the more it became my main priority.

I became so pedantic about every aspect of my life. *I'd better not have a glass of wine tonight because that might affect our chances … I'd better not have too much of that food because it might make me too acidic.* I went from being a fairly easy-going, good person to be around to being a complete stress-head about everything.

As a couple, all you want to do is be close and supportive of one another at a time like this. Yet my husband must have been thinking, *Why can't you just back off, for goodness sake? There's more to life than just this.* But there isn't more to life than 'just this' when you're the woman and you think time is running out.

Can we fix it?

If something is wrong, I'm the sort of person who wants to find a way to fix it. My husband probably would have been happy to carry on trying for the next two or three years. But one year had already passed and I saw the clock ticking. I wanted to try IVF.

When we saw the director of the IVF clinic it became quite apparent that this wasn't something that could just 'be fixed'. It was a process that was going to be lengthy, and it was going to be costly, and it was going to be emotional.

My husband was surprised by what was involved, and at that point he did think twice about it. One of his major concerns was that someone might recognise him at the clinic, as he was rather well known in our community.

Looking back, we probably didn't discuss it fully. Quite selfishly, it was all about me. 'You don't have to go through this,' I told him. 'But I'd really like it if you would.' I assured him it would be discreet, and I would help protect his identity. He agreed to do it – pretty much just to placate me.

To start the process, we needed to have some tests done. And it transpired that I had chlamydia. My first thoughts were: *How can I have picked this up? Has my husband been unfaithful to me?*

As much as my husband reassured me he hadn't been unfaithful, until I had confirmation of his results, I couldn't rest. In the end, his test came back negative. That was a relief. But I felt awful then, to think that I was the one who had possibly jeopardised our chances of having children. And he then suggested I might have been playing around on him. It certainly made our relationship tense.

That tension eased a little when someone from the clinic explained that the testing procedures were sometimes inaccurate, and that there was always the chance of a false negative result.

The doctor said the chlamydia had probably been in my system for a long time, and it may have caused internal scarring. I chastised myself for everything I'd ever done that might have caused this problem. Then I thought, *Surely I'm not the only person in the world who's had more than one partner. How come none of my other girlfriends have ever had to go through this?*

We were then tested for a whole suite of sexually transmitted diseases (as the clinic couldn't store cells that might carry anything communicable). Waiting for the results seemed to take forever. Since one unexpected thing had already occurred, I couldn't help wondering whether anything else might crop up.

All of this was really destructive emotionally. It did nothing to put my mind in the right place for falling pregnant.

More tests

The STD tests were all clear. Time for more tests. I had an HSG (an X-ray of the uterus and fallopian tubes taken after a dye is inserted). I found that hideously painful and vowed I would never go through any testing procedures again. Of course, within a couple of days I'd forgotten about the pain and all I wanted to do was get a result. I would have gone through anything to achieve my goal.

So I had a laparoscopy. It revealed a lot of scarring, particularly around my right ovary and fallopian tube. The specialist couldn't say that that had definitely been the cause of our problems, but it couldn't have helped the situation. In any case, it was able to be cleared. But the specialist said, 'Chances are, the scarring will return. You really have to get on with the program now. You have to take it seriously.'

'Believe me, I'm taking this seriously!' I said.

The pressure was on even more than it had been. I started on some fertility drugs, realising that I would need to undergo a full IVF procedure if the drugs didn't have any effect.

Knowing that my husband and I had a boat, the specialist advised me to go out on the water for a few days and 'have some fun'. He encouraged me to laugh and relax; even to have a few wines. I wanted to take his advice, but I wasn't sure if I could. *How are you supposed to relax when this is on your mind?* I thought.

We actually did go out and moor up the boat for the night, and a very bizarre thing happened. Getting up in the morning and walking up onto the deck, I spotted another boat moored about 100 metres away. The owner was clearly visible to me. Of all people, it was our specialist. I rushed back down under the deck and said, 'I can't go back up there – he's going to know what we're doing!'

Despite taking the fertility drugs (and going out on the boat) nothing happened. So it was time for our first IVF cycle. When it finally came around, I was full of hope. The specialist had told us there was no good reason why we couldn't conceive. So I was absolutely sure it was going to work.

The flip side of IVF

While the IVF gave me hope, it also made me feel like a bit of a loser. I didn't know anyone else who had had fertility problems or IVF, so I felt quite alone.

> So it was time for our first IVF cycle. When it finally came around, I was full of hope.

I also had the sense that people were constantly feeling sorry for me. Even the lady at pathology who took my blood sample felt sorry for me. It was nice that people were supportive, but it made me feel self-conscious. *I don't want your sympathy. I just want this thing to happen!* I thought.

One day at the IVF clinic, someone recognised my husband. 'That was the last thing I needed,' he told me. He was pretty good about it, but he also asked whether he could avoid coming to the clinic if he didn't have to.

It didn't worry me that I had to go there alone (even to deliver his semen sample). Because at the time I really thought it was all my fault. *He didn't ask for this*, I thought. It was all about me wanting a baby. And as the woman, I thought my body was responsible for not producing the goods.

Finally the day arrived when I received the results from our first IVF cycle.

'Anna*, we have some news. Sadly, this cycle has not produced a pregnancy for you.'

I had been so sure we would be getting good news, so it was heart wrenching to hear those words. I had a terrible feeling in the pit of my stomach and I wasn't sure whether I wanted to vomit or not. I asked the lady from the clinic to repeat what she had said, just to be sure.

When I told my husband, he was very rational about it. 'We've only had one go. What did you expect?' he asked me.

That started off the whole it's-all-right-for-you conversation. 'Are you taking this as seriously as I am?' I asked.

Underneath my show of anger, I actually felt like a real failure. As a woman, I couldn't do the job that I was put on this planet to do.

The IVF process had been hard. The whole thing had been a series of needles. I had needles in my cervix. I had needles in my tummy. And I felt like I'd been to that pathology lab so many times. The thought of repeating all of that filled me with trepidation. For a split second I wondered, *Do I really want to do that again?* But the answer came back swiftly – *Nothing is more important than having a child.*

I was determined to do whatever I could until I got the result I wanted.

Take a break

I was keen to get on with the next IVF cycle ASAP. But with Christmas approaching, we couldn't start it until the end of January.

Once again the doctor advised me to go out on our boat, have some fun and enjoy the holiday season. I remember thinking, *That is so frivolous! I can't do anything proactive for six weeks. This is going to destroy my Christmas.*

Everyone was on go-slow. It was holidays, beach, and more holidays for everyone around me. That was completely frustrating. If I have a project, it isn't natural for me to just drop it for a period of time.

I couldn't just do nothing. So I went to see an acupuncturist and I threw myself into the pilates classes I had recently joined. Maybe these sorts of activities provide stress relief for some people. But not for me. Just by being there, my mind was focused on the end result. It was about me trying to control this thing I couldn't control.

I'd also heard about a renowned herbalist who had helped many couples to conceive. I couldn't get an appointment for months, but I was able to fill out an online survey and order some herbs on the Internet. I remember thinking that it might be the answer to my prayers. A slight sense of relief came with that.

In the lead-up to Christmas, I wasn't really in party mode, but I gradually softened on that point.

I had been so careful with everything I had eaten and drunk for such a long time. The thought of going through the festive season watching everyone around me 'troughing' into everything while I abstained wasn't very appealing. *I need a bloomin' break*, I decided. *I need a little bit of lightheartedness in my life.*

I was really looking forward to our New Year's Eve party. I decided it would be nice to have a few drinks. In fact, it would be downright annoying to be pregnant that night!

Things weren't all hunky dory, but I definitely relaxed a bit more during that time. I also stopped having sex according to all the charts and indicators, and forgot all about ovulation dates. Our sex life had been too mechanical for too long, so it was a relief for some spontaneity to come back into it.

Of course, the holidays did eventually come to an end. Finally! Now I just had to wait for my period to arrive so I could get on with the next IVF cycle. It seemed to be taking a long time though. Very odd indeed. So by early February I thought I would get it checked out by my GP.

My GP rang me after the appointment.

'Anna, I don't know how to tell you this. I'm so thrilled for you … You're pregnant!'

I nearly fell over. 'Can you say that again?' I beamed.

She gently warned me to keep my feet on the ground, but nothing could stop the euphoria that came over me in that moment.

Funnily enough, the herbs I had ordered arrived that same day. I felt that was quite symbolic. Similar things have happened to me in a number of situations, actually; I toil away, trying every possible avenue I can to fix a situation, and then right at the end a solution or answer comes along as if to say, 'It could have been this easy all along! You didn't have to take the hard road'.

Anyway, I worked out that we must have conceived on day ten of my cycle. All that time I thought I had been ovulating later than that.

Counting the days of your cycle and taking your temperature … you do all these things with the best intentions. But just because there are guidelines that fit the majority of the population, they don't fit everybody. So that was quite a lesson for me. Maybe we should have left it to nature to work it all out. What a revelation! After about fifteen months of trying everything and anything, it happened when I wasn't even on the case.

My pregnancy

I don't want my story to end there. I don't want to give the false impression that things were 'happily ever after' from the moment of conception.

During my pregnancy, I just did not rest. I would wake up in the middle of the night and think, *Wow, there's a baby inside me … But what if it doesn't last?*

I was completely paranoid about every morsel of food and drink I put into my body. I wanted to wrap myself up in cotton wool.

My being so paranoid and neurotic can't have been easy for the people around me, especially my husband. We had gone through all the stress of conceiving to arrive at this pregnancy – and even more stress.

> Sitting up at the computer one night at 10 p.m., my waters broke. *Is this for real?* I wondered.

Everything went well until week twenty-six, when I ended up in hospital for a week with an impacted uterus. I had to lie on my back and not go anywhere or do anything until the uterus moved into the correct position. I told myself, *Whatever happens, I can cope.* Because that's what I do, I cope.

I obeyed the doctor's orders to go home and take it easy. Nevertheless, my little girl arrived at week 34 because of yet another complication – an incompetent cervix. Sitting up at the computer one night at 10 p.m., my waters broke. *Is this for real?* I wondered. Thankfully, being the organised person I am, I had my bags packed and ready.

My daughter was in special care for the first ten days of her life. She was born with two club feet as well, so she needed a splint on one of her legs. So nothing was easy for us! But it didn't matter, as it was such a joyful time.

While we absolutely adored her, the first few months of her life were a challenge. She was really tiny and needed a lot of feeding. She didn't sleep well. We also went through daily physiotherapy to fix her feet. Then there were a few nasty viruses going around and we were warned to keep her away from anyone who might be unwell. So she was this incredibly precious little bundle. My husband found that quite tough. My body had been so precious while we'd been trying to get pregnant, and then while I carried the baby. And now I was consumed with concerns for this premature baby. It never seemed to end.

A second child

Both my husband and I grew up with a sibling, and I always wanted the same for my daughter.

I didn't consider trying for a second child until my daughter was about fifteen months old. It had been a rough couple of years, and I didn't actually feel ready for another baby. But my GP and my gynaecologist suggested that if I wanted another one I should get on with it as soon as possible. A lot of our friends had had children in quick succession, so it seemed like a normal thing to do.

I knew that the problems we'd had with our first baby had put a lot of pressure on our marriage. So I was a bit nervous that a second child might create even more of an issue. But I'd become pretty selfish by that point. I thought, *It's now or never, and I can't face 'never'.*

My husband wasn't at all convinced. He could see that having two little ones was going to be hard work. But nonetheless, I decided that we should start trying again.

Slipping back into control mode, I decided to get my body super receptive to pregnancy. I saw my acupuncturist again and also started taking a herbal tonic from a Chinese medicine practitioner.

My day-to-day life was pretty hectic at that time. I was looking after a child who wasn't sleeping well, our marriage was struggling, and we were building a new house.

Yet my mindset was quite different from the first time we'd tried to conceive. I felt blessed that I'd been able to have one child. If I couldn't fall pregnant, there wasn't the sense that it would destroy my life. A second baby would be a bonus, but it wasn't absolutely essential to my future happiness.

Within a few months, I was pregnant. It was quite a shock, because I hadn't expected it to happen so soon. It was all fine until I took the tests for Down syndrome. My risk rate was 1 in 51, so I ended up having an amniocentesis. Sure enough, the results came back to confirm I was carrying a Down syndrome baby.

I think out of this whole process, that was the toughest point. I did lots of crying.

My husband and I had talked about this scenario in the past. We had always felt it wouldn't be responsible for us to bring a child into the world in these circumstances. A few physical and mental problems are associated with this condition, so we didn't feel it was the thing for us to do – for the child's sake as well as ours. We were older parents, and the child was likely to outlive us. I didn't think it was fair to put that pressure on our daughter either.

Of course, when you're actually faced with a decision like this, it's not as easy as saying, 'Well, that's what we've said in the past so that's what we'll do.'

We took a few days to consider it, but in the end we decided to terminate the pregnancy. Because the pregnancy was further along, I actually had to deliver the baby. It was 24 hours of very painful labour. The most difficult thing my husband has ever had to endure was watching me go through that.

In the end we were given a choice about whether we would see the baby or not. We both decided to see her – and to name her Chloe. The nurses put her in a little dress and I held her briefly. They also prepared a little book with her hand prints and footprints for us. We organised for her ashes to be scattered at the hospital's Garden of Remembrance which we could visit any time.

In the week that followed, I went through some harrowing emotions. I kept looking at my daughter and feeling so lucky to have her. But it didn't make up for what I thought I had done. It just didn't sit well with me.

There was also overwhelming disappointment. I thought, *Why is God doing this to us? We just want to be good, dedicated parents.*

My husband was worrying about me. He pretty much wanted to shake me and say, 'Pull yourself together.' I construed that as his not understanding what I was going through.

I had some grief counselling after the termination. To my surprise, I ended up speaking more about my relationship than I did about the loss of our baby.

My husband was suffering from the aftermath of a difficult first year with our baby girl. Then, to have another trauma was too much for him, especially since he hadn't been that enthusiastic about having another child in the first place. I was feeling quite alone in my needs and desires.

Try again?

We had been through such a lot of heartache that my husband said to me, 'Do we really want to go through all of that again?' I was wondering the same thing myself. Although I believed the chances of another disability showing up were quite low, I knew it probably made more sense to stick with one child and avoid any more emotional challenges.

But there was an urge in me I couldn't seem to ignore. I thought I would never be happy unless I had tried everything I could to have two children. I couldn't stand the thought of my daughter asking me one day, 'Why don't I have a brother or sister?' I wanted to be able to tell her with complete honesty that I had tried everything I could to make that possible.

So I decided to leave it all to fate. *If it happens, it happens. If it doesn't, then it isn't meant to be.*

My husband and I weren't getting along too well. But one night we attended a party with lots of old friends and felt close for the first time in quite a while. We actually conceived that night, four months after we began trying.

I had another tricky pregnancy, but in the end another beautiful girl came into our lives.

Double-edged sword

I honestly would not trade parenthood for anything. Even though we went through a lot, I've always felt very blessed to have one child, let alone two. And that will never go away. However, I fully recognise the pressure it put on our relationship. I don't think I saw that as it was all happening. But I do see it now.

Very recently I discovered that my husband was having an affair. When he explained why he'd done it, he reflected a lot on the years just past. From his perspective, everything was a drama. He found me very overbearing about the whole children thing. I was almost removed from the relationship because I was so focused on falling pregnant, and then so focused on the babies.

I can really see it from the man's point of view now. They don't get the same amount of attention they're used to getting. You're not the same person, because you're so wrapped up in this whole thing. Rightly or wrongly, it contributed massively to the breakdown of our marriage – and eventually to our separation.

Fortunately, our separation was brief, and we have reunited now. We've both had a chance to understand what really went on during the past few years – and that has helped us to understand one another a lot better. So I think in the long run this whole experience will contribute to us becoming a lot stronger as a couple and a lot more intuitive about each other's feelings.

I'm hoping and believing that I'm going to turn around in ten years' time and say, 'Okay, that was a huge struggle, and it highlighted the deficiencies in our relationship, but we've come out the other side and we're all a whole lot better for it.'

So what could I have done differently back then? I can now see that it isn't worth pushing a man into fatherhood before he is ready. If you do that, you have to be prepared for the fact that it may be the making or breaking of your relationship. And I think that, basically, we could have benefited from knowing the importance of just being in love, enjoying life and enjoying each other.

* Real names were replaced with pseudonyms in this story.

Sophia's story

UP TO THE AGE OF 30, I'D LIVED A CHARMED LIFE. MY PARENTS emigrated from Hong Kong and they're together to this day. I worked hard at school, went to university, met my husband and worked in a couple of satisfying jobs. Everything went smoothly, and I had no reason to expect it would ever be any other way.

Andrew* and I had been married for about five years when we decided to have our first baby. Conception was no problem – I got pregnant within about four months. I just assumed everything would be fine, as it always had been.

But when I was about seven weeks' pregnant, something happened that would turn my world upside down for years to come.

It was a Sunday. Andrew was away fishing and I was home alone. When I went to the bathroom, I noticed some spotting on my underpants. *This can't be good*, I thought, and I started to panic. I felt even worse when I couldn't reach Andrew on his mobile phone.

So I called a doctor for some advice. 'You're not cramping, so it might be fine. Just get some rest,' he told me.

Although I returned to bed for the rest of the day, the bleeding became heavier. So the next day I went to see a doctor in person. Right there in the doctor's office, I started to have stomach cramps. A feeling of dread, panic and loss of control rose from deep inside me. It was clear that I was miscarrying, so I was rushed to the emergency department of a nearby hospital. I kept thinking, *Maybe if I don't panic, I won't really have a miscarriage.* But it was pretty hard to stop that sense of panic from taking over.

In my mind I had pictured the next chapter of our lives together as three. But now we had lost our baby. The whole event came as a complete shock to me. I was devastated. I couldn't help blaming myself. So many questions went through my mind. Was I working too hard? Was I running around too much?

I had some tests done after that, to see if there was a medical explanation for the miscarriage. The results were fine. 'Bad luck, try again,' they said. So with my confidence shaken, that's what we set out to do.

Trying again

After a few months of irregular periods, there was no sign of a baby. So I started a course of traditional Chinese medicine and acupuncture. I hoped it would help me fall pregnant and I hoped that it would help sustain the pregnancy.

While I was doing these practical things to fall pregnant, my life situation wasn't really all that conducive to conception. My husband had just started working in Asia. I was flying back and forth between continents to be with him, and then coming home to see my elderly parents. The commuting was stressful, and our lives felt unsettled. There was no sense of a 'nest' for this little family we were trying to create.

> The commuting was stressful, and our lives felt unsettled. There was no sense of a 'nest' for this little family we were trying to create.

Since I was out of my home country for long periods of time, I couldn't see my Chinese medicine practitioner regularly. She gave me herbs in bulk to take back to Asia with me, but she wasn't able to continually adapt a program to suit my changing needs.

After a year or so, I also enlisted the help of a GP. He suggested clomid (a fertility drug) might help give my body a bit of a kick along. Lo and behold, I fell pregnant immediately.

My first thought was: *Oh my God, I just have to make it through the first twelve weeks.* I imagined that twelve-week mark would be a magical moment after which I would feel safe again.

I didn't enjoy that pregnancy for a second. I was constantly expecting something bad to happen. Every time I'd go to the loo, I'd check for signs of blood. *Hang in there*, I told the baby – but the statement was full of fear.

At eleven weeks, my worst fear came true. There I was, so close to the twelve-week mark, and I miscarried. It felt incredibly cruel. I was far more shattered than I had been with the first miscarriage. It felt as if those eleven weeks of constant worry, fear and being so careful all came to nothing.

Again, I found myself flying back and forth between countries – this time for more tests. I found out that my hormone levels were low, but they were still within the band considered 'normal', so we didn't have a definitive answer. In some ways that was worse, since there was nothing that could be 'fixed'.

> I didn't enjoy that pregnancy for a second. I was constantly expecting something bad to happen.

I went into a deep depression for a few months. I even thought about ending my life. I contemplated what method I would use – I worked out, in detail, the most efficient and painless way to end it all.

The thing that stopped me from taking those thoughts further was my parents. I knew it would destroy them if I did something like that.

In the end, a book called *Miscarriage*, by Lesley Regan, saved me. It made me look beyond my current situation and into the future. Most importantly, it gave me hope. And that hope was enough to bring me out of the darkness.

My sole focus

My parents passed on a strong work ethic to me. *If you work at something, you'll get it.* That had always been true in my life. So where could I turn to now that my body seemed incapable of doing what I wanted it to do? I had a ridiculous amount of time on my hands to ponder this question. While my husband worked in Asia, I didn't have a work permit. So basically I could play golf and do yoga, or think about trying to get pregnant. It was in my face all day long.

I peed on a lot of sticks during that time. I peed on sticks to see when I was ovulating and I peed on sticks to see if I was pregnant. It meant that I could hardly think about anything else, really.

I'm a very proactive person. Since it was taking so long to fall pregnant again, I was in constant contact with doctors, having tests and discussing various options for assisted conception.

> Fortunately, someone entered my life to shift my focus and make things quite a bit easier … a pet dog.

With each new thing I would try, I would convince myself that this time it was going to work. But gradually it dawned on me that I wasn't going to get pregnant that easily. I felt a sense of failure, a sense of unfairness, a deep sadness and emptiness.

Because of my irregular periods, the doctors thought it might be helpful to track my egg's cycle with an ultrasound and perform an artificial insemination at the time of ovulation. They performed this procedure twice. It involved having extra hormone injections in my stomach to boost my egg production. I hate needles so the whole thing was pretty stressful.

During one of the scans, some endometriosis showed up. The doctors said not to worry about it; it would disappear once I fell pregnant. But I couldn't help being spooked by the knowledge it was there – it felt like one more reason I mightn't be able to have a baby. One more way my body was letting me down.

A new friend

Fortunately, someone entered my life to shift my focus and make things quite a bit easier … a pet dog. I regularly stopped by the pet shop in our local shopping mall and Lulu was always there. She was a gorgeous little thing, but as more time went on, I noticed her becoming quite listless. In the end my husband and I decided to give her a life outside the glass box she had been confined to for nine months.

It took a lot of energy and dedication to revive Lulu's personality and energy. I spent lots of time with her, and bit by bit she came back. For the first time in ages, I stopped focusing on myself. Lulu needed me, and that felt good. I needed her too.

More high tech

In time, we decided to try IVF. We flew back home to attend a clinic with a high success rate. It cost us a lot of money. So I couldn't help thinking: *This has to work.* Andrew really thought this would be the final solution. We would have our baby at last.

> In time, we decided to try IVF. We flew back home to attend a clinic with a high success rate. It cost us a lot of money. So I couldn't help thinking: *This has to work.*

In the end they only harvested three eggs, and only one embryo was good enough to implant.

I was in the car with Andrew on the day they rang through the results. As we drove through a busy junction, I heard the news that the embryo hadn't taken. I tried not to cry; I wanted to be strong for Andrew. When I looked over at him, I saw he was close to tears as well.

'We can try again,' he told me. But both of us knew our hearts weren't ready to be ripped out again. We had invested so much in this process, emotionally and financially. In some ways it felt like having a miscarriage, without getting pregnant first.

Even today, I can't drive past that same junction without feeling immense sadness and a sense of loss.

I decided I needed to take a break from IVF. I wanted to give my body a chance to become clear of all the chemicals before we contemplated going through the whole process again.

The doctor said we could return to IVF at a later date, but he warned us that it mightn't be all that straightforward. 'Your egg production is low,' he said. 'So you might reach a point where you need to consider egg donation.' I was devastated by this prospect. But I tried to reassure myself by thinking: *At least it would still be Andrew's baby.*

I returned to a course of Chinese medicine and acupuncture. The remedies were supposed to prepare my body, slowly, for a pregnancy. Despite everything the doctors had told me, I still hoped that this low-tech option might give me a chance of conceiving naturally. And if not, I believed it would get my body into the best possible condition for another IVF attempt.

Alternatives

Andrew and I were determined to have a couple of children, and that meant we were happy to adopt if we couldn't conceive. The thing is, by this stage we were heading for our mid-thirties. We understood that the chances of being selected as adoptive parents would decrease as we got older. Because of this time pressure, we started the process for adopting a baby from China.

Adoption felt like a great option, but I still wanted to give myself the best chance possible of falling pregnant. We continued walking on these two paths, hoping that one way or another we might become parents soon.

I instinctively knew that it wasn't just my body that was stopping me from falling pregnant. I suspected my fertility was also being affected by a psychological block. Every time I would do a pregnancy test, of course I was so let down to see the negative result. But somewhere deep down, there was also a sense of relief. *At least I won't have to spend the next twelve weeks worrying about another miscarriage,* I would think.

> Every time I would do a pregnancy test, of course I was so let down to see the negative result. But somewhere deep down, there was also a sense of relief.

The idea of miscarrying again, and spiralling into those dark emotions, still had a grip on me – although it was mainly at a subconscious level. I quickly buried any conscious thoughts along those lines.

Around that time, I read about a clinical psychologist and hypnotherapist who specialised in fertility. She had a really high success rate, so I booked in for an appointment.

This lady seemed upbeat about my chances of conceiving naturally. So I told her about the endometriosis. And my hormone levels. And everything else. She still seemed optimistic. *Clearly this woman doesn't understand my situation!* I thought.

I had some pretty big issues with my body. I was really angry with it. I felt it had let me down.

We embarked on a series of sessions to purge all of the emotional baggage I had about falling pregnant. The counselling part of my sessions helped me to work through any issues that I was conscious of, and the hypnosis helped me to uncover issues on a subconscious level.

Until then, I hadn't spoken with anyone about my miscarriages. I don't have any sisters, and with my mum in her seventies, well, I was afraid that her blood pressure would go up if she had to worry about my problems on top of her own.

I had some pretty big issues with my body. I was really angry with it. I felt it had let me down. I was convinced that if I fell pregnant, I would miscarry again. With this therapist's help, I realised I could change that viewpoint, and I started talking about my body – and to my body – in a positive way. I even started to say some affirmations every night before bed. *I am super fertile. My body is strong and healthy. I can easily and happily have a healthy and happy baby.*

She also got me to release some beliefs I had about being too old to conceive. I had heard that when you hit 35 your fertility nosedived. I'd heard it so many times that I truly believed it. (And I'd just hit 35, by the way!) But with some hypnotherapy – as well as hearing stories about many of my doctor's 'older' clients who had conceived – I quickly came to realise that my age wasn't a definitive barrier to conception.

I also discussed the troublesome aspects of my relationship with my parents. I had always felt that my mother favoured my brother over me. I believed that if I needed her help, she wouldn't be there for me. But during my therapy I realised that I had helped to create this situation. My brother had been quite dependent on my mother, while I had always looked after myself. I realised that all I needed to do was learn to ask for help – and it would be there. I felt much happier, and much more supported, once I had gained that insight.

> Alkl of these processes started to have a profound effect on the way my mind worked ... I became a lot calmer.

I did a lot of guided visualisations during the hypnotherapy. During one session, I imagined myself packing all of my issues into a box and throwing them over the edge of a boat. In another session, I saw myself pregnant and talking to my baby. I let myself experience all of the love I felt for this little person.

All of these processes started to have a profound effect on the way my mind worked in everyday life. I became a lot calmer. I learnt not to hold onto things, and not to go over and over an issue in my mind. I brought my thoughts back to the broader picture, rather than getting stuck in the small stuff. So when a car would cut me off on the road, or when somebody pushed in front of me in a queue, it no longer felt like the end of the world!

It also changed the way I looked at difficult issues. We were in the middle of a renovation at that time, and one night our ceiling came down. Instead of stressing about it, I decided just to laugh. That definitely made me see how much my view of the world had changed.

I was only seeing the hypnotherapist for about two months when I noticed that my periods had become regular.

With the adoption process unfolding faster than expected, and the prospect of a natural conception due to the work I was doing on myself,

I knew everything was going to work out okay. *One way or another, I will have a baby by next year.* As a result, we weren't trying quite so desperately to conceive.

I also started to relax more in general. I had been off alcohol for five years in an attempt to make my body ready for a baby. But in the lead-up to Christmas, I thought, *Sod it!*, and had a few social drinks.

All of this coincided with the completion of our renovation. After years of commuting between countries, followed by living in an unfinished house, finally Andrew and I were living together in a place that truly felt like a family home.

Endings and beginnings

One day in the bathroom I found myself doing yet another pregnancy test. But this time it was positive. I sat down on the loo, lost for words. I had been waiting for that moment every day for the three years that had passed since my second miscarriage.

When I called Andrew at work, he was beside himself. He screamed down the phone, 'Oh my God!'

We were basically on the cusp of adopting a child, so the timing was incredible.

> After months of connecting with my baby boy in utero, I finally got to meet my son, James, in person; the most wonderful moment of my life.

I rang my hypnotherapist to tell her the good news. She was very happy for me, and said, 'You've worked hard, and this is what I expected to happen.' Her attitude was really nice, reinforcing the idea that I was more than capable of conceiving and carrying a baby.

Because of the hypnotherapy, I could really enjoy the pregnancy. It felt completely different from my earlier pregnancies. I was so happy and relaxed. I knew it would all be fine, and it was.

After months of connecting with my baby boy in utero, I finally got to meet my son, James, in person; the most wonderful moment of my life. It was like meeting an old friend again. I felt I already knew him so well.

Number two

I made a great group of friends in my antenatal classes. We all stayed in contact after having our babies. Most of us wanted to have more children at some stage. *Oh God, I bet I'll be the last one to fall pregnant*, I thought.

My GP suggested I use birth control, which seemed ridiculous after it took a total of five years to have James. Given my age, I was worried about leaving it too much longer before having another baby. I went back to see my hypnotherapist to chat about it all. She reminded me that my age was no problem, and suggested that only I would know when the time was right to have my next child.

I really enjoyed the first year of motherhood, but I definitely wasn't ready for another child immediately. Every time I would bend down to pick up James out of the bath, I would think: *I can't have a second baby yet, how could I pick James up if I was heavily pregnant?*

Then, one day, James finished his bath and stood up by himself. Lifting him up was so much easier. And right then, I knew I was ready to bring another baby into our home.

Andrew was travelling for his work that month, so we only had sex once that cycle. Yet I fell pregnant. Incredibly, I was the first one in my antenatal group to conceive the second time around.

Treasuring my babies

When baby Robert arrived in the world, it really felt like the last part of my healing process. A couple of years ago, it would have been extremely confronting to talk about my miscarriages. But now I have my two healthy sons, it feels like Andrew and I are the luckiest people in the world.

I actually believe I'm a better mum now than if I'd had a baby right at the beginning of all of this. Because of everything I've been through, I treasure them all the more. I'm so happy to be at home with my boys, and I don't want to miss a minute of this experience, even if I am ready to pass out by the time I put them to bed.

Even Lulu loves the boys. These days she likes to lie under Robert's cot as if she's protecting him while he sleeps.

I couldn't ask for anything more.

Real names were replaced with pseudonyms in this story.

Megan's story

M Y PARTNER, JUSTIN*, COMES FROM A CONSERVATIVE CATHOLIC family. Before our marriage, we did the taboo thing and lived together. There wasn't any overt conflict with Justin's parents, but they did have a few quiet words with him about it. We felt like the black sheep of the family. When they visited us from out of town, they never stayed with us in our apartment. I assumed I was the 'wrong kind of girl' for their son.

The next chapter

At 33, the wedding bells finally rang. The ceremony took place in an old, deserted church in a small coastal town. We had to get special permission to use the venue, and we filled it with yellow native flowers.

The next adventure – parenthood. That felt like the natural progression. I had always expected it would happen that way, and I couldn't wait to be a mum.

I stopped taking the pill not long after we married. Justin was happy for me to do that when I felt ready. So, from the start, I was running the show.

The first six months during which we tried to conceive were uneventful. I had heard it could take a while, so even as the months ticked by, I wasn't worried. But gradually I became more and more disappointed each time I would get my period.

My instinctive reaction was to do some research. I read up on ovulation, temperature charts, and what to look for on each day of your cycle. Now aware of the intricacies of the reproductive process, I realised that the odds of a sperm and egg actually meeting and doing their job were so long, any conception would be a miracle.

The clinical approach

I switched from a romantic approach to a very scientific one. I took my temperature every morning and recorded all of the data on changes in my body. Our sex lives became more clinical.

With my new scientific approach, I was well and truly controlling the process. Surely that would mean I would have more luck? Apparently not. Another six, seven, eight, nine months rolled by and still nothing happened.

My whole existence seemed to revolve around which day I was up to in my cycle. Once each period finished, I would be waiting for the fertile period. Nervous. Hopeful. Ever watchful for signs of ovulation. Then I would count down the days until my period was due, tuning into the tiniest sensations in my body, wondering whether they were signs of pregnancy.

> My whole existence seemed to revolve around which day I was up to in my cycle.

I did a lot of pregnancy tests. They were always negative, but every time I would wonder if the test had been faulty. I developed a real mistrust of those things!

I became obsessed; a mad woman on a mission. It must have been unbearable for Justin, but we didn't communicate about it – he just went along with everything I told him. There was only one occasion when he mentioned that he was finding anything difficult: he didn't like it when I insisted, 'Now is the time we have to have sex.' I could have guessed that for myself. His body language intimated that it had all become a bit too mechanical.

My in-laws are family people. Justin's parents love grandchildren being born. And there was no shortage of them coming from Justin's siblings. There were five under the age of five to be exact. I knew I was being irrational, and I certainly didn't consciously want to take away their happiness, but it was so hard to be around them, smack bang in the face of their joy. I avoided contact with them as much as I could.

One day my brother-in-law told me the others were finding it hard. They thought that they had done something wrong. I fell silent when he told me that. Processing what he said, I could see that I was being unfair to them. *But I can't change how I feel*, I told myself.

After fifteen months, I went to see a gynaecologist. An investigative procedure revealed a tiny fibroid in my uterus, although it wasn't big enough to cause fertility issues.

Justin was also tested. A few sperm were irregular in shape, but overall his sample was fine.

I spoke with the gynaecologist about the possibility of in vitro fertilisation. I had always assumed that I could fall back on IVF if we had trouble conceiving. Now it was looking like a good option. I didn't feel as though I could trust my body to do its job any more, so I liked the idea of getting assistance from some capable people.

> I told her we had been having trouble conceiving, and she blatantly asked, 'Have you looked into IVF?'

I didn't jump straight into IVF. Being in a senior position at work, I wasn't sure if I would be able to get time off work for appointments and procedures. On top of that, I happened to be working at a Catholic school. There was a big moral debate in the media about IVF at that time, and I was strongly aware that many members of the Catholic Church didn't support this technology. I assumed my boss would be opposed to the idea.

Being a straight-talking lady, my boss happened to ask me when I would be having children. I told her we had been having trouble conceiving, and she blatantly asked, 'Have you looked into IVF?' I was stunned by her acceptance of the process. What's more, she said it would be fine for me to take time off from work if I decided to go ahead with it. That was actually the impetus for me to begin IVF.

I wouldn't have dreamed of telling my in-laws what we were embarking on. Given their religious background, I thought they would be dead against it. I also wondered what they thought about the absence of children in our lives. Perhaps they assumed it had been a conscious decision, driven by me, the ambitious woman focused on career rather than family. If only they knew the truth – that becoming a mother meant everything to me.

It felt as though I was never going to fall pregnant. And I had no idea what I would do with my life if I didn't have children. It wasn't something I had ever considered. I had friends who had consciously decided not to have kids, and they seemed to enjoy a lot of travelling. I guessedthat would be what I would do, too. But there had to be more to life than travel … I just couldn't work out what else there could be.

IVF begins

About eighteen months after we first started trying, we found ourselves sitting in the office of an IVF specialist. I had brought along all of my temperature charts from the last year or so, keen to show him the data I had diligently gathered.

He looked at me and said, 'Can I just tell you one thing? Stop taking your bloody temperature.'

Justin blurted out, 'Thank God you said that!'

I felt relieved. I wouldn't have to do all that hard work any more, as I had an expert telling me I didn't have to.

Another doctor explained the IVF process to us. She said, 'Since there is nothing wrong with either of you, you will conceive at some stage, whether naturally or on IVF.' She then went through the stats, showing us that our chances of falling pregnant with IVF were higher, per cycle, than trying to conceive on our own. That sounded good to me. I was sick of waiting for this to happen. At the end of the appointment I clapped my hands and said, 'Right. Let's go!'

I felt incredibly optimistic. And so empowered! I had troops to support me in achieving this goal. And I was paying for it – surely that would add to a sense of guarantee?

The whole IVF process felt like a blur. Before work I would head to the clinic to line up with other women waiting for injections. The clinic was crammed into a small building, and the waiting room was always filled to capacity on those mornings. Women rushed in on their way to work, suited up and business-like. No-one looked each other in the eye. It was all heads down in magazines until your name was called – and then the rush out the door to get to work on time.

When the treatments began, it felt like we were keeping a sinister secret from Justin's family. But I thought it was only a matter of time before we would be successful, so I didn't think we would have to keep it a secret for too long.

> The whole IVF process felt like a blur. Before work I would head to the clinic to line up with other women waiting for injections.

Then came the day I found out the results of my first IVF cycle. We had been told the mathematical chances of falling pregnant each cycle. I tried to be realistic. I tried to prepare myself for the worst scenario. However, there was a deeply ingrained, irrational belief that this was going to work. When I was told that it hadn't, I was devastated.

Justin did what he normally does in difficult situations. He kept quiet and busied himself with practical tasks. We were renovating our house, so there was always something that needed to be done.

Out of the darkness – briefly

I was home alone when the IVF nurse called with the results of my second IVF cycle.

'Congratulations. You've got a positive result,' she said.

I can't remember how I told Justin, but we were both elated. We shared the news with both of our families straightaway. They were so excited, chatting away about their future grandchild. Mum bought a pair of baby booties the following day, and Justin's mum began to make a beautifully embroidered baby blanket.

Bad news

At eight weeks we went along for a scan. The doctor pointed out all sorts of things on the screen. I was mesmerised.

'Just looking for the heartbeat now,' he said, followed by a long pause.

'Still looking for the heartbeat,' he said. Another pause.

'Sometimes it's hard to pick up,' he said, and relocated me to another room where I was hooked up to a super-duper machine that should definitely be able to find the heartbeat.

> That night I lay in the bath … For those few moments I felt safe; hidden away from the world and its harsh realities.

But the new machine couldn't track it down either. The doctor knew straightaway. There was no life in this tiny foetus. I don't remember how he told us, but I do remember how I felt. Like I'd been hit with a sledge-hammer.

They moved us into a small room with a couple of chairs, a little round table and a box of tissues. The 'bad news' room. I couldn't get any words out. Just heaving sobs. *I'm living my worst nightmare*, I thought. Justin was in shock. There was nothing either of us could say. We just sat close, with our hands on each other's knees.

I called my mum when I got home.

'Mum …' I said, all choked up.

That's all I needed to say. She knew straightaway. She listened to me cry, and offered me reassuring words every now and then.

'You'll get through this. It will make you stronger,' she assured me.

That night I lay in the bath. I remember submerging my whole body, head and all, under the warm water. For those few moments I felt safe; hidden away from the world and its harsh realities.

I went into hospital for a curette to remove the foetus. I felt incredibly fragile and in need of Justin's support and love. He was pretty shut down that day. During the procedure he decided to head back to work, to attend to the practical tasks he knew he could control.

As I lay there in recovery, I felt so alone.

I felt a real mess heading into the next IVF cycle. I was in grief about the miscarriage, felt anger towards Justin, and had a sense of hopelessness about our seemingly endless battle to conceive. Justin told me to pull myself together, which was the worst thing he could have said. I suppose he was just trying to be practical. He didn't want either of us to wallow in misery any longer than necessary.

Justin didn't want any counselling, but I knew I couldn't cope without it.

I spoke with the clinic's counsellor about Justin leaving me at the hospital. That single event triggered so many feelings that had long been bottled up. It brought up anger I had towards my own father. Mum and Dad had separated when I was young, and from then on he was never around. He never took an interest in me, and he let me down many, many times.

> Before all of this, our relationship was relaxed and fun. But now, not much fun was being had.

It was helpful to have the chance to vent some emotional baggage. But I really should have dealt with all of these issues long before starting IVF.

Even though he didn't want counselling, Justin was going through a hard time of his own. Our relationship had been through so much in the past two years, and he had struggled with my intense personality shift. Before all of this, our relationship was relaxed and fun. But now, not much fun was being had.

Justin blamed himself a lot for the fertility problems. He was very athletic and healthy, and always took pride in his physical strength. Being on the IVF program probably shook his confidence. But I never bothered to find out about that. I was completely self-centred.

I often talked about conception and IVF. But it was always a one-way conversation. I would relay information to him, without letting him do any talking or questioning. I felt convinced I was doing what was best for both of us.

Round three

I went into the third IVF cycle carrying a weight of grief. I'd had a rude awakening from my earlier optimism. The IVF now felt like an impossible mission. It would take nothing short of a miracle to get me pregnant, I was convinced of that.

> The IVF now felt like an impossible mission. It would take nothing short of a miracle to get me pregnant.

Work was stressful. Even though my life had been turned upside down, I would front up every day, act professional and pretend everything was fine. The pretending was the hardest part.

When the embryo didn't take, I was beside myself. I marched into the doctor's office and demanded that he start injecting me immediately for the next cycle.

'You have to give your body a rest,' he said.

He suggested that I should slow down the IVF process. Take a break. Justin panicked, asking the doctor if it was doing any damage to my body. 'No, she's physically very strong. It's her emotions I'm concerned about,' he said.

With that feedback about my physical condition, I was happy to push on.

However, something had to change in my life, because I was overwhelmed. I took leave from my job. As usual, I drove the decision. I didn't consult Justin about the impact that this would have on our finances or anything else. I assumed I was doing what was best for both of us.

Being without work made things worse. I felt aimless – and even more focused on falling pregnant.

I got a call from my mother-in-law around that time. She gently asked how things were going, and then she said, 'Have you given IVF some thought?'

The implication was clear – IVF was okay with her. I revealed everything that had been happening.

'I thought you might have trouble coming to terms with it because of the church's views,' I told her.

'My religion is important to me,' Judy said. 'But when it comes to decisions like this, I make up my own mind.'

From that moment on, my in-laws could not have been more supportive. Judy was fantastic. I felt a huge shift just knowing I had her on side.

> ... Judy asked me how Justin was coping. I was completely taken aback ... He had the easy part!

At one stage Judy asked me how Justin was coping. I was completely taken aback. It hadn't even occurred to me that he would have anything to cope with. He had the easy part in all this! I was the one carrying the burden.

Judy must have sensed that I was feeling alone in my efforts to have a baby. She sensitively assured me that even though Justin mightn't express it in words, he really was with me on this journey. She knew first-hand what it felt like, because Justin's dad was much the same – a loving man, who didn't always communicate his emotions.

That whole conversation gave me a good jolt. I started to be more considerate of Justin from then on.

My fourth and fifth cycles passed by with no luck, and I genuinely thought I wasn't going to have a successful outcome with IVF. But things were changing for me on another level. This wall I'd had around me was coming down. I was letting in love and support from family members. That definitely made things easier.

Justin was relieved that our IVF experiences were finally out in the open. Even though he didn't openly communicate about difficult things with his family, they were very close. It made a big difference for him to have their support.

The fifth cycle represented a noticeable turning point. I started injecting at home, and that took a fair bit of pressure out of the equation. No more lining up at the clinic early in the morning.

I also realised that I needed to get back into the workforce. So I took a teaching job at a school where no-one knew me. Where no-one asked me questions. It felt much better being occupied by some new experiences. And it wasn't a high-level job, so I felt no pressure to be a 'superwoman'.

> A nurse rang me after that sixth cycle with some unexpected news. I was pregnant.

Our last go?

Given the structure of government funding for IVF at the time, I believed that we could only really afford to have six cycles of IVF. The cost would go right up after that. So the sixth cycle was going to be my Russian roulette. My last shot. *I'm running out of time.*

I wondered whether I should have a break before that final cycle. A conversation with my mum influenced me a lot. All of this love oozed out of her. 'Don't give up. You can do this,' she told me.

Mum accompanied me to my next appointment. I'd been to a lot of them on my own so it felt good to have her there.

The specialist said he could put me on a lower level of medical intervention for the next cycle. He explained that the government subsidies for this type of treatment could continue for any number of cycles. I let out a sigh of relief.

I went ahead with that sixth cycle, just as Mum suggested. Thank God it wasn't my last chance.

A nurse rang me after that sixth cycle with some unexpected news. I was pregnant.

I went to Justin's office to tell him in person. I found him working at his computer.

'Guess what? It worked!' I told him.

He paused for a moment. Excitement spread across his face. Then he looked back at his computer and visibly composed himself. I guessed what he must have been thinking. *We can't afford to get too caught up in this. It only makes it worse when we fall.*

We were both cautious about telling people this time around. We didn't want to share the news before the first scan. Justin's parents were diplomatic – they didn't ask for an update during that time, waiting instead for us to deliver any good or bad news we might have.

> Justin was just as engrossed in the pregnancy as I was. We had a whole new relationship from then on.

It was impossible to keep the news from my mum. I don't recall ever telling her I was pregnant. She just knew.

Our eight-week scan was a totally different experience this time. I cried with happiness as we saw our healthy baby, and heard its heart beating. Justin was deeply relieved. He squeezed my hand.

Soon after, we went to a birthday party with Justin's family. Justin told his five-year-old niece that she could announce to everyone that we would be having a baby. She proudly strutted into the kitchen where Judy and a few others were washing and drying dishes. 'Megan and Justin are having a baby,' she said.

The whole room stiffened. You could almost hear what everyone was thinking. *Dear God, what has this child said?*

Then they saw me smiling. Everyone started jumping up and down and screaming.

My new obsession

I loved being pregnant. It gave me a whole new obsession. I read a lot about pregnancy and birth, probably no different from many first-time mums. Justin was just as engrossed in the pregnancy as I was. We had a whole new relationship from then on. They were much happier times.

There were a few problems with the pregnancy though. Perhaps because of the pregnancy hormones, my tiny fibroid was no longer tiny. It set off contractions 25 weeks into the pregnancy (a bit past halfway), and I ended up in hospital for a week. That whole episode plunged me back into doubt about my body's capabilities.

By 38 weeks, I was so nervous about the birth. I didn't trust myself to deliver this baby safely. My body hadn't been able to do anything without medical intervention, and I was sure this would be no different. The doctor agreed to do a caesarean section on the day of my 38-week appointment. Justin hopped on his bike and pedalled as fast as he could to meet me at the hospital.

I felt so glad that everyone around me was controlling the birth. And after a few minutes, the doctor was holding up our baby girl. I had tried not to think about which gender I would prefer, but the fact that it was a girl made that moment even more special for me. I fed her immediately and shed a few tears. I was unbelievably relieved to get through that whole difficult chapter with a happy ending.

Justin was besotted with his new daughter. He used to stare at her in a hypnotic way, and sing to her for hours. He would look up at me and say, 'Thank you so much.'

From a distance, Justin's dad had watched us endure everything. He was particularly overwhelmed when he met our baby girl. 'Thank you so much for bringing this happiness into our family,' he said to me from his heart. Since he's a man of few words, I understood the weight of his sentiment.

I was so pleased to have Olivia in our lives that I didn't even contemplate having more children. She was a miracle.

We were the happiest people we knew. We had climbed to the top of a mountain. It took a long time to calm down from that elation. In fact, it is still with me today.

Doing it the natural way

Three months after the birth, I had an operation to remove the fibroid from my uterus.

Three more months passed, and I realised I hadn't had a period for a while. I went to the GP to find out what was going on. She got me to do a pregnancy test.

> My faith in my own body had been restored a little.

A few minutes later, we were looking at a positive result. After all we'd been through, and after having no faith in my body whatsoever, how was this even possible? I cried as I sat with my GP and told her everything we'd been through. She checked the result again and with a smile said, 'Yes, confirmed! You are definitely up the duff.' I laughed.

Ten weeks into my pregnancy, I miscarried. Back to the hospital for a curette. It felt completely different this time. Justin was there constantly, and he kept holding Olivia close to me. 'Look how lucky we are,' he would say.

Even though I'd miscarried, it felt like this baby's conception had been another miracle in our lives. My faith in my own body had been restored a little.

When we told Justin's parents that we had conceived naturally, Judy suggested that Justin's faith in his body would have been restored as well.

A couple of months later, the same thing happened. No period. A visit to the GP's office. Even now, there was no way I could trust those pesky home pregnancy tests!

Once more, she confirmed I was pregnant. I laughed with disbelief. I couldn't even remember having sex in the previous month! It felt like a joke that things could swing around so much; that this could happen so easily.

I had a wonderful pregnancy, and Justin and I were thrilled to bring another daughter, Annabel, home from the hospital with us.

Another miracle?

When Annabel was eleven months old, I found myself at the GP's office yet again. I discovered that I was pregnant, this time at age forty-one. My jaw dropped, and I couldn't stop giggling.

I left there feeling quite smug. *Look at how clever I am.*

I immediately took my two girls to see Justin, who was busy renovating our new house. He was standing there with a hammer in his hand as I asked him, 'Do you think the house looks big enough?'

'Looks big enough to me,' he said.

'Big enough for three kids?' I asked him.

'Bloody hell,' he said. He dropped the hammer. But he was smiling.

Our third child, a rotund, blue-eyed, shiny-faced boy called Alex, was born by c-section eight months later.

The doctor conducted a tubal ligation immediately after the birth, to attend to my contraceptive needs from then on. In my mid-thirties I thought I was never going to fall pregnant. Now here I was at the other end of the spectrum, having my tubes tied.

Looking back

In the years we tried to conceive our first baby, I made life pretty hard for myself, and for those around me. With the benefit of hindsight, I can see that things had to get worse before they could get better. From the grief of my miscarriage came the need for a new way of operating. Justin and I opened up to the support of family members who would have been there for us much earlier, if we had let them. As I softened towards those loved ones, I softened towards myself. I made changes in my lifestyle to better nurture my spirit. And I finally started to consider Justin's feelings.

We were in a completely different state of mind when we conceived our second and third children. I was no longer blinkered by my conception obsession. Justin and I were a team. We loved being parents together. We were so grateful for what we had.

Although we struggle with the daily grind and pressures of family life, we are extremely proud of our family and we are constantly aware of how fortunate we are.

Real names were replaced with pseudonyms in this story.

Beth's story

13

WE WERE SURROUNDED by GOOD FRIENDS AS IT TURNED midnight on New Year's Eve. Time for everyone to make a wish. I can't remember whether I said it aloud, or just in my own head. I wished that I could have a child.

Nick* and I had been together for twelve years, and he didn't want to have children. I had agreed with him up until now. But at the age of 35, something changed for me. I really wanted to be a mum. I had the sense that life with a child would be full of joy and expansive possibilities.

Now I had a dilemma on my hands.

The most tearful twelve months of my life began. Conversation after conversation about whether or not to have a baby. Sometimes holding hands, often in tears, covering the same ground over and over again. I desperately wanted a child and Nick didn't.

Nick is a deep thinker, and his reservations had lots of layers. How could he be a good father *and* continue to be an artist? Didn't parenthood mean a boring life in suburbia, with no opportunity to travel or chase our dreams? Would he face the same predicament as his own mother – and have his career stopped short by having children?

Nick was also deeply concerned about overpopulation; the human race gobbling up the earth's resources in an unsustainable way. Could we really justify bringing another human being to the planet, given the damage that we do? This issue played on my mind a lot too, but I thought there must be a way we could bring up a child while staying true to our ethics and values.

'I'm only talking about one child here, Nick,' I reassured him. I felt that was the best compromise between my desire to have children and our concerns about the planet.

In a way, I didn't take Nick's fears all that seriously. I strongly believed he would be a fantastic father – and anyone who knew him well thought the same thing. Couldn't we just get on with it?

During our many discussions, we came up with possible ways we could have a child and still look after both of our needs. I could be the primary caregiver so that Nick's career wouldn't be compromised. We could still travel and go on adventures – we would just take our child with us. We went into quite a lot of detail, even down to the finances. Maybe all this analysis made things more complicated than they needed to be. At least it set the scene for us to be mindful of each other's practical needs.

It felt like we were climbing a mountain. Bit by bit, we trekked up the side of that mountain, feeling exhausted by the amount of planning and communication and emotions involved, and having no idea what we would see when we arrived at the summit.

I was consumed by a lot of fear during this time. Every time I had to raise the issue with Nick, I felt frightened. Deep down, I feared that he wouldn't love me if I pushed the issue too hard. Bracing myself to talk to him always felt like I was about to leap across a large crevice with my eyes tightly shut.

I also experienced a lot of helplessness. A lot of feeling stuck. I wondered, *Will Nick and I ever see eye to eye on this issue? Why does this have to be so difficult? Everyone else seems to have partners who want children.*

There was also a deep well of sadness about the whole situation.

Whenever I felt sad, I would do a meditation. I had been studying Buddhism, and I began a practice which allowed me to experience my own pain and suffering with an intention that it might save other human beings from experiencing the same. It wasn't about being a martyr. It was about believing that some good could come of these difficult times. In my meditations, I would focus on transforming my sadness into something else. I would breathe out white light, and the intention for other people to have happiness and joy and babies.

My Buddhist studies reminded me to treat Nick with kindness and compassion. I tried not to bring up the baby topic if I was coming from emotions of anger or frustration. But often I just wished he'd get over it! I'm sure he wanted me to get over it as well.

> Where possible, we would have our baby discussions over a cup of tea and cake somewhere special.

Where possible, we would have our baby discussions over a cup of tea and cake somewhere special. One of our chats took place in a café overlooking a beautiful nature reserve. We used it as an opportunity to connect and, in a sense, enjoy ourselves, rather than having awkward conversations while washing the dishes at home.

After a year of talking and crying, there was nothing more to be said. Gridlock. That prompted us to get help from someone on the outside – a family therapist. A friend recommended a male therapist, and I thought that would be ideal. I didn't want to end up with a female, or any therapist who would sympathise with my side of the story just because wanting children was the cultural norm. I wanted Nick to feel understood, and I wanted the process to be fair.

The therapist broached a question we had been avoiding: if we couldn't resolve this issue, would we go our separate ways? In facing that option in the safe environment of a therapist's office, it actually confirmed for Nick and I how special our relationship was, and how much we didn't want to lose each other. The therapist also pointed out to Nick that if he ended up with a new partner, this same dilemma might reappear for him.

We went out for a beautiful lunch after that session. We didn't do any more analysis. It felt right to give it some space. Perhaps it was symbolic that we were going to stick together and get through this.

After all those discussions, and a big nudge from the therapist, we finally reached a decision. Nick cautiously agreed that it would be okay for me to go off the pill and see what happened.

Off the pill

Off the pill at last! I felt so much excitement at the possibility of falling pregnant. I had a belief that maybe it would happen really fast. So much hope.

But there was still this sense that falling pregnant was my agenda, and not Nick's. I didn't want to push him too hard – I thought we needed some time to let things settle. I never insisted on making love at a certain time in order to make a baby. As a result, we had a very hit-and-miss approach in our efforts to conceive.

After a year, I went to see a naturopath. I wanted to create the optimal physical conditions for a pregnancy, and naturopathy seemed like a good way to achieve that.

The naturopath recommended that I take my temperature to check if I was ovulating properly. So every morning I would get the thermometer out as I lay in bed. Nick and I may have stopped our endless discussions about it, but the thermometer reminded him that this wasn't just something that was on the backburner. We both felt very awkward for those few moments each morning.

A friend recommended I see an acupuncturist. Since acupuncture works with the body's energy, I thought it would be a good adjunct to the naturopathy. It was also another way to ensure I was doing all I could to set the right conditions for conception and pregnancy.

Still I didn't fall pregnant. Sometimes I would get disappointed that it wasn't happening. I would imagine how beautiful it would be to carry a baby inside me and bring it into the world. At other times I would feel relieved that it wasn't happening. The more time I gave it, the more time Nick would have to get used to the idea. Patient. Impatient. Excited. Sad. Sometimes all in the same day. My mood was completely changeable!

After about eighteen months, a GP suggested that I see a fertility specialist. My periods had been regular, and my temperature charts indicated that I had been ovulating. But I still wanted to make sure that there wasn't anything wrong with my body. So off I went to see the specialist.

I hadn't even thought about the fact that the specialist would want to involve Nick in the process. Oh dear. He needed to provide a semen sample.

Suddenly I had to face my fears about involving Nick in everything. We had no choice but to communicate about the biological realities of conception. It was a blessing in a way, because Nick amazed me with his helpfulness, and we became more of a team.

> Suddenly I had to face my fears about involving Nick in everything. We had no choice but to communicate about the biological realities of conception.

Our test results were all fine, so our fertility issues were officially 'unexplained'. It was good to know everything was in working order. But it felt as though another question mark was added to a growing list of unknowns. (The biggest unknown of all was whether we would even have a baby at the end of all of this.)

I only saw the specialist to find out if there were any problems. But he started to tell me about some options that might help us conceive. Nick and I didn't feel particularly comfortable with the idea of assisted conception, but we allowed ourselves to be swept along with this new approach for a while, dutifully doing everything we were told to do. If we didn't end up having a child, at least I would know that I had tried everything I could to make it happen. That felt very important to me.

There was a sense of panic in the medical model about how quickly you should try to get pregnant. But my intuition told me that rushing things wasn't going to help our situation. We needed lots of space and time. So even though we went through a series of treatments one after the other, I never bought into any high expectations, nor a sense of urgency.

To start with, I took the fertility drug, clomid, to help stimulate ovulation. Then we had sex at the times we were supposed to. Over the four cycles of clomid, my period took longer and longer to arrive each time. The doctor was intrigued by the way my body had slowed down, as he hadn't seen that happen before. (Looking back, it was quite symbolic of our mindset towards conceiving.)

One night, when we were due to have intercourse, we had a guest staying in our house. With such thin walls, the idea of doing it at home was unappealing. We decided to pack a picnic and head to the hills for a romantic evening. We managed to find a secluded spot. On finishing our meal, it was time to do the deed when, out of nowhere, a pack of wild dogs surrounded us, barking ferociously. We had no choice but to pack up and run. Very much a case of 'This wasn't meant to be'.

Next, we tried three rounds of intrauterine insemination (IUI). This is the procedure that used to be known as artificial insemination, and it's often one of the first assisted conception treatments offered to couples with 'unexplained infertility'. Still no pregnancy.

That year went by in a blur. It felt like I was standing on a travelator – the type you see in airports. It was all happening around me as I went along complying with everything I was instructed to do.

Nick came on board, providing semen samples and being fantastic about it all. But it still felt like he was doing all of this for me. I knew he was relieved that I wasn't falling pregnant.

On the recommendation of my naturopath, I saw a kinesiologist. (Kinesiology uses muscle tests to identify imbalances in the body's energy, from which to identify the body's healing needs.) I thought this would be just one more thing to try, along with naturopathy, acupuncture and medical assistance, to ensure that I had done everything I possibly could. It was helpful, because the kinesiologist got me to address my anxieties about bringing a child into an overpopulated world. She helped me to see that my child could contribute to the world, which felt quite different from my previous fear that an extra human being might ravage the planet!

We quietly bowed out of our medical expedition after twelve months. IVF was the next logical step, but we knew from the start that that option didn't feel right for us.

> Turning 40 felt quite symbolic. I knew I had to start adjusting to the reality that we probably wouldn't have a child.

Nick must have thought to himself, *Phew*.

Left to our own resources

When we stopped seeing the fertility specialist, we believed the odds were against us conceiving. But I thought to myself, *You never know.* I continued taking folate, just in case. And after sex, I continued my habit of lying still for a while, in case that improved the odds of the sperm getting to their destination.

We looked into the possibility of adoption. I really liked the idea of providing a loving family for a child from overseas, but I worried about making Nick jump through a myriad of administrative hoops, given his ambivalence to having children in the first place.

Even so, we attended a seminar to find out more about overseas adoption. We discovered that our ages would prevent us from being eligible. So that wasn't to be. But we went along to the seminar as a couple, and in some ways that occasion cemented our relationship.

Turning 40 felt quite symbolic. I knew I had to start adjusting to the reality that we probably wouldn't have a child. My fortieth birthday party was an outdoor picnic with a group of friends. On the surface I was celebrating this milestone in my life, but really it felt like I was just going through the motions. I socialised and smiled. But the same sad thought kept crossing my mind: *I'm never going to have a child.*

With babies off the agenda, Nick and I started to reconnect as a couple without that huge question mark hanging over us the whole time. We started making love more often.

A special Christmas

A year and a half after we'd finished our fertility treatments, I went back to see my GP for a pap smear. I can't remember exactly what she said to me, but she must have asked all the right questions. I had a few tears and told her how sad I was that I hadn't been able to have a child. She gently suggested that I could book in for some grief counselling with a lady who worked in the same premises. She had a waiting list, but if I put my name down, I might be able to see her after Christmas.

I decided to book in to see the counsellor, because I knew I needed to come to terms with things. I already had the sense that everything was going to be okay; we'd done our best and it just wasn't meant to be. But I still didn't have a really strong picture of what life would be like without a child, and I knew I needed to do something about that.

When the Christmas break began, Nick and I headed off for a camping trip. We did an advanced trek around a cliff face which posed all sorts of challenges and risks. We nearly ran out of water one day, and had to come up with an improvised way to fix Nick's hiking boot the next. Our teamwork was first class.

We went directly from our camping trip to my parents' farm. We spent Christmas there, on the beautiful piece of land where I grew up. I remember sitting on the couch holding Nick's hand, crying as I told Mum and Dad that we'd given up our attempts to conceive. My sadness had turned into grief. And one of the reasons I was grieving was because my parents would never have a grandchild.

Our time in my family home was very special. Everyone was relaxed and I had a few drinks for the first time in ages. A highlight of the trip was walking out through the paddocks to inspect a part of the land that Mum and Dad were regenerating with native trees and plants. It was such a joy to see all of this unexpected life returning to the land; somehow the birds and wildlife had found their way to this new patch of wilderness.

On Christmas night, Nick and I made love. I got up straightaway instead of lying still afterwards. I wanted to sit and meditate. There was nothing all that remarkable about the meditation. But for some reason I didn't have that sense of grasping for the unobtainable that I'd been filled with every time I had made love with Nick in the past four years.

> We scooted out to buy a new test, and the result was the same. I was pregnant.

When we got home from our holiday, my period was a couple of days late. I didn't feel any different, but I thought I may as well use up the one last pregnancy test that was sitting in the cupboard. It was past its expiry date, so I wasn't even sure if it would work properly.

The test turned pink. Hmmm. It wasn't supposed to do that. I found Nick and told him, 'I've done this test. It's out of date so it's probably not even right, but it's saying that I could be pregnant.'

He went pale, but then he said, 'I'm so happy for you, darling.' Some people might interpret that as a bad thing, but I thought it was precious.

We scooted out to buy a new test, and the result was the same. I was pregnant.

Our baby boy

I felt incredibly lucky. But I wondered if there might be more lessons ahead for me. I didn't want to take anything for granted and I worried a lot about miscarrying. I was so anxious leading up to our first scan that I had diarrhoea. But everything was fine. It was amazing to see this baby had a brain and a heart and everything else it needed.

We tried really hard not to get into the baby consumerist culture. Where possible, we bought secondhand things. And we came up with a number of ways to minimise our baby's impact on the environment.

Our baby boy arrived on Father's Day. It felt like a miracle – the perfect gift for Nick. He had been so unsure about it all, even throughout the pregnancy. But the moment he held his son – this little person who looked identical to him – a beautiful sense of calm came over him. From that day on he became the wonderful father I always knew he would be.

We stuck to the plans we had made all those years ago. I became the primary caregiver, and Nick continued with his work full time. We've travelled and had lots of adventures with our little fellow in tow.

I'm now juggling work and motherhood, and still trying to work out how to cope with it all. But our son is a huge blessing in our lives, and an amazing little person. In some ways this is the unknown summit we were climbing towards a few years ago. And there are still plenty of unknown summits ahead. Will we be able to move around and live in different places, and still find decent schools for our son? How will it be when he is twenty and we're in our early sixties?

My son's conception still feels like a mystery to me. There were so many things that came together at the time he was conceived, on both an emotional and a spiritual level. I don't claim to have any of the answers. But I do know that, for me, it felt right to try everything I could to make it happen. And I realise that there was also a time when letting go was helpful too. I had to draw a line somewhere and say 'no more'. No more alternative therapies. No more medical assistance. Otherwise I could have gone on endlessly spending money and making life awful for Nick and me.

Perhaps our little boy was waiting for us to experience this journey. To grow stronger in our relationship and within ourselves. Perhaps he knew when the time was right. Maybe he had a connection with my family and the place where he was conceived. Or maybe he needed a natural conception rather than a medical one, for whatever reason. It reminds me of a Buddhist quote: 'Nothing ever exists entirely alone; everything is in relation to everything else.'

* *Real names were replaced with pseudonyms in this story.*

14

Janet's story

THERE IS ONE THING THE CONCEPTION OF EACH OF MY BABIES HAS in common. I was laughing while we were having sex.

We conceived our first child after two years and two months of trying. I was over the whole sex-to-a-timetable thing. *Just get on with it and then I'll read a book*, I remember thinking. During sex I started to laugh about the whole scenario. Trevor said, 'You know, you're not helping.' I thought that was really funny, so I laughed even harder.

It took eighteen months to conceive our second child. I was cracking up over something when that happened, too. And it was great sex. *This is the kind of sex where you should conceive*, I thought.

There aren't many common threads in my two conception stories, apart from that laughter.

The making of Conor

I focused a lot on my body during my first journey to conception. I never thought it would be easy to achieve a pregnancy. A doctor had diagnosed me with PCOS in my early twenties – that's polycystic ovary syndrome. It affects women in different ways. For me, I didn't ovulate every month, and my periods were irregular.

'You're going to need drugs to conceive,' they told me. *Surely it's not going to be that hard*, I thought. I knew it might take a relatively long time to conceive, but I decided I would rather take time than take drugs.

I wasn't against drugs per se, more the idea of going straight for the quick-fix option. I wanted to conceive when I was healthy and my body was ready, not by forcing my body to accept a pregnancy through chemical manipulation.

Long before I tried to conceive, I shopped around countless practitioners to see who could help me with the PCOS. Eventually I found a naturopath who specialised in hormone issues. I felt better within days of seeing her.

I discovered that you can also manage PCOS with a healthy diet and weight management. So when Trevor and I decided to have a baby, I ate well and lost some weight. My naturopath continued to provide me with herbs and eventually some flower essences.

I figured that in the months I did ovulate, we would just try to 'catch the egg'. I charted my menstrual cycle, learning to read the changes in my body throughout the month. It didn't take long to work out when I was in the fertile zone.

After about eight months of trying to conceive, Trevor and I went to Ireland. I joked with him, 'You have to knock me up when we're there.'

We fell in love with the place. Even thinking about it now, I wish I was back there.

We conceived during that magical trip. I knew I must have been pregnant because I was tired and slightly nauseous and I had sore breasts. But my excitement was short-lived. Lying in bed one night, I realised that the little life in me had snuffed out. I just felt it stop. And I thought, *Oh, God, that was a shift*. There was no immediate bleeding, but in the next couple of days the signs of pregnancy faded. Deep down I knew it was over – even though I didn't want to believe it was.

Four or five months later, it happened again. Even as we were having sex I thought, *I know that sensation. I'm pregnant*. But the next day I started bleeding. Another miscarriage.

Trevor and I were deeply sad both times I miscarried. I remember that second time he bought me a bunch of apricot roses.

I had moments of anger. *It's not fucking fair*, I thought. *I'm going to stay in bed and cry and eat chocolate!* But neither of us had the terrible grief some couples experience. Once the emotions had run their course, we got on with our business.

After the second miscarriage I rang my naturopath to discuss what had happened and to alter my remedies accordingly. I also ramped up my healthy eating.

My naturopath suggested that acupuncture may have further benefits for me. And it definitely did. My periods became a lot more regular thanks to weekly acupuncture treatments.

Trevor supported me in everything I was doing to improve our chances of conceiving. Thankfully, the fertility issues didn't come between us. We both wanted a baby – and that united us.

Pregnant friends

When you're having a difficult fertility journey, there are lots of opportunities to make a choice about how you're going to feel and how you're going to deal with it. While we were trying to conceive, many of Trevor's friends were getting pregnant.

Personally, I don't think it's fair to get cranky about other people's journeys or experiences just because you perceive theirs to be easier – you can't know what they're going through.

> Trevor supported me in everything I was doing to improve our chances of conceiving ... We both wanted a baby – and that united us.

I could have chosen to be joyful for those friends, or I could have chosen to wallow in my own distress. I decided to go for the first option. I used to crochet baby rugs for those couples and, in time, I also worked away at my own baby rug.

Subconscious blocks

I did a good job getting my body ready for conception and pregnancy. But looking back now, I can see another layer – a lot of stuff on an emotional level – that probably contributed to the infertility in some way.

My mother had terminal cancer the whole time Trevor and I were trying. On many occasions I sat in her lounge room drinking tea and making small talk. She always sat in a rocking chair in the corner. She didn't want to be hugged. She didn't want to talk about the cancer, let alone the prospect of death. I wanted to be there for her. I wanted to help her come to terms with it. But when I asked her about the cancer she didn't want to talk about it. When I didn't ask, she thought I didn't care.

It consumed a lot of emotional energy, and that probably didn't help my physical health.

In retrospect, I didn't have enough room for both a child and a terminally ill mother at the one time.

I probably had to see Mum off the planet before I had a child. In retrospect, I didn't have enough room for both a child and a terminally ill mother at the one time.

Just after Mum died, I found a book by Niravi Payne called *The Whole Person Fertility Program*. It prompted me to write down my family's attitudes towards children. You should have seen the stuff I came up with! The whole time I had been trying to conceive, I had actually harboured fears about falling pregnant and bringing a child into the world. I hadn't even known these beliefs were there, tucked away in my subconscious.

Children are inconvenient and difficult and they slow you down. Being an adult is really hard. Being a parent is a horrendous occupation. My mother did a good job raising me, but through her words and actions, she had subtly conveyed these attitudes. Somewhere along the line I had absorbed them. But the moment I wrote them down, I was free. I could see that I didn't actually agree with any of them.

Almost directly after that process, I fell pregnant. Obviously other pivotal changes had occurred, both on a physical and an emotional level, before it happened. I couldn't attribute it to any one factor. I believe it was a combination of everything.

Finally!

I achieved this pregnancy after 26 long months. I felt the physical signs of pregnancy, but this time I refused to believe it was happening. I was in complete denial.

My infertility had become this self-perpetuating entity – this thing I had become familiar with. It was a comfort zone and I wasn't sure I was ready to say goodbye to it, as illogical as that may sound.

> My infertility had become this self-perpetuating entity – this thing I had become familiar with.

Seeing how tired I was, a friend said, 'I bet you're pregnant.'

'I bet the value of your mortgage payment that I'm not,' I told her, my denial in full swing.

Eventually I weed on a stick. It was one of those moments you never forget. Standing in our ensuite, waiting for the result to show up, with Trevor on the phone. 'I'm not pregnant. I'm not pregnant,' I told him as we waited.

Then I said, 'There's a result.'

'Yes?' he asked.

'Oh, my God, it's positive!'

'Right, okay,' he said, in his usual laconic tone.

I could almost hear his mind ticking away, processing what I had just said. *I'm going to be a father. Holy shit!*

I went into a spiral of hysteria. *Oh, my God. Oh, my God.*

I burst into my bedroom, lay on my bed and called a few friends. We screamed at each other and it was fabulous.

I wasn't worried about miscarrying this time. Somehow, I knew it would be fine.

The birth

During my first pregnancy, I planned a home birth. A birth is something most of us cherish for the rest of our lives. It was really important to me that my baby and I had the best, most gentle experience possible. The more I read about hospital practices, the more I felt my decision was sound.

Just as planned, I had Trevor, a friend and a midwife by my side for the labour and it was all going beautifully. But after about 24 hours the midwife thought the baby was stuck. On her recommendation, I was transferred to the hospital for a caesarean.

Before the operation, an obstetrician came to examine me. Someone who I had never seen before in my life. Can you take back the words 'being raped.' Then it happened. She shoved her hand into me so hard that I screamed. I told her to take it out of my body, but she didn't. It felt as though I was being raped.

Conor was born in an operation that lasted only a few minutes. After the procedure, they wheeled me away to a recovery area. They refused to admit Conor to that part of the hospital.

'Please take me to my child,' I said repeatedly. But two hours passed before that happened.

I felt an overwhelming urgency to see him. I kept watching my vital signs on the monitors around me. My blood pressure was normal. My oxygen levels were normal. There was nothing wrong with me.

Thankfully Conor was in his father's arms, skin on skin, for those precious first hours of his life. But it was barbaric of them to separate him from me like that. I will never get that time back.

I really struggled after that. I had post-traumatic stress disorder from the whole experience, but it took a while to recognise just how serious things were.

For the first few months of Conor's life, I just muddled my way through things and did what needed to be done for him. I breastfed him a lot, and gave him lots of cuddles. But those moments were often truncated by flashbacks to the hospital. I often struggled to go back to sleep after giving Conor a night feed. I would lie there with scenes from the hospital looping over and over in my mind.

After six months, the stress hit a peak.

One day it suddenly occurred to me that I could end it all. I didn't have to live like this. I didn't have to live with the pain and my child didn't have to have this fucked up, angry mother who was distressed all the time and wasn't coping. For the first time in my life I considered suicide. Fortunately there was a part of my brain which was like a running Zen commentary. It said: *You know, it's not really normal to think like this. You might want to do something about it.*

I rang Trevor at work and said, 'You should come home – *now*.'

From that point on I got help.

Trevor took time off work and stayed home with me. It was obviously difficult for him having a partner who was suicidal and stricken with grief. But he was loving, patient and completely understanding through it all.

> One day it occurred to me that I could end it all ... For the first time in my life I considered suicide

When Trev went back to work, women I knew would come over and babysit me for the day and see that I was okay.

I had some talking therapy with a woman who specialised in birth issues. She had been a birth attendant for 30 years and she really 'got it'. I came away from those sessions no longer suicidal.

For a long while after, I was still depressed, and still suffering from post-traumatic stress. I took some natural remedies to help with that, and continued to get support from Trevor and my friends.

I kept wondering: *If I have another baby how can I stop all of this from happening again?*

Often with post-traumatic stress disorder, you fantasise about ways to save yourself if the traumatic event ever happens again. What you're really doing is trying to save yourself from what happened the first time, which is obviously impossible.

Part of my effort to save myself, and others, from the same type of trauma, was establishing an online community. I recognised the lack of support for women who had had a home birth transfer, or just a traumatic hospital birth, and I needed to create my own support group. I also had a strong urge to promote home birth. I built a website, and women gathered in this cyberspace to share their own birth experiences. In time, we all started to get together in person as well.

> While I was grateful to have one child in my life, that didn't make the longing for a second child any easier to handle.

Trying to conceive again

In the thick of my recovery, we actually started trying for another baby. *I've got nothing to lose here*, I convinced myself. *It will probably take a while anyway.* Maybe on a subconscious level, I thought it would give me something to think about other than post-traumatic stress.

Trying to conceive definitely gave me something else to think about. But it also gave me something else to stress about – on top of everything else.

To my surprise, the second journey was kind of like a continuation of the first one. I didn't start off thinking, *This is a nice fresh start.* It was more like: *Oh, my God, it takes me forever to conceive!* I was in that old mindset straightaway.

While I was grateful to have one child in my life, that didn't make the longing for a second child any easier to handle.

Fortunately I had more support this time around. The first time, I didn't really talk about it with anyone. I didn't want to be a watched pot, and I didn't want to hear any clichéd advice. But now I had lots of friends who had kids. In particular, I had a very dear friend who had had her own difficulties conceiving. She really understood, and that was excellent.

My issues around Conor's birth definitely impacted on our efforts to conceive.

Having sex was really complex. For many months, I had terrible flashbacks to what had happened in hospital. Trevor understood what I was experiencing, and he remained patient and loving.

The grief around Conor's birth had become self-perpetuating, and it was difficult to know how to live without it. I didn't really want to live without it either. It was one of the few tangible reminders of his birth that belonged to me. It sucked. But it belonged to me.

One afternoon I spoke to a friend who helped me see I was choosing to hold onto my pain and grief. When that awareness came to me, it was a major turning point. I consciously decided to let the pain and grief go.

Not too long after that, my sister fell pregnant. I was pleased for her, but it brought up a lot of stuff for me. Until then, I hadn't realised the extent of my distress about Conor being taken away from me. I called a friend and she gave me the space to just talk and let it unravel. I fell to the floor and cried and cried about how they had taken him away and how afraid I was that I mightn't be able to protect another baby. Such a powerful emotional afternoon. My friend stayed on the phone through it all.

> I was finally able to invest in a new journey towards birth. It felt like a fresh start.

I was finally able to invest in a new journey towards birth. It felt like a fresh start. I owed that to myself and to my baby.

Towards a joyous birth

There was no actual day I found out about my pregnancy with Isobel. One weekend I said to Trev, 'I feel weird. I have fatigue, heartburn and nausea. I think I'm pregnant!' I suddenly remembered feeling very similar things at the start of my pregnancy with Conor.

I didn't do a test. I decided to just sit with the inner knowing of being pregnant. It felt very gentle to embrace the pregnancy without having that definite marker which says, 'You are pregnant from this moment on'. I started telling friends about two weeks later, at Conor's second birthday party.

The party was held in a park. At one stage I was sitting next to Trevor and I said, 'You know, we really are having a baby!' And we shared a beautiful hug.

A few weeks into the pregnancy, I rang a midwife and asked her to take me on as a client. Then I got on with life, enjoying being pregnant and being a mother to Conor.

Every time I felt this little person move inside me, I was transfixed. Nothing else in the universe seemed to matter. *My God! That was an elbow!* I enjoyed that connection with my new baby just as much as I had when I was pregnant with Conor.

At 37 weeks my midwife pulled out. I made the decision then to free birth my baby, which was just as well since I woke up the next morning in labour!

> Every time I felt this little person move inside me I was transfixed. Nothing else in the universe seemed to matter.

It was 50 hours of strong, active, hard-to-ignore labour. Trevor was wonderful – even more so than the first time around, because there wasn't a midwife there. I was the expert this time so all he had to do was be supportive. A dear friend and a doula (birth support person) also stayed for my whole labour.

After giving birth to Isobel, I ended up transferring to hospital to get some stitches. But I was very feisty and I was also high on endorphins, so all that empowered me. I made sure I was treated well.

Of course the story doesn't end there. Now I'm raising my two kids and I absolutely love it. I still have a mild version of post-traumatic stress, but life is so much easier than it was in those first few months after Conor's birth.

Maybe we'll try to have another baby again one day. If that happens, I'll at least know that we've done it twice before. Hopefully, I'll drop the idea that it takes me forever to conceive. I did learn to create a fresh journey towards birth. Maybe I can learn to create a fresh journey towards conception too.

Postscript: Janet conceived her third child, quite by surprise, after being interviewed for this book.

Jonathan's story

I'M 49. AFTER BEING SINGLE FOR A LONG TIME, ALONG COMES Katrina*. She is this wonderful 35-year-old woman who is well travelled and seems to share the same values as I have. We have a business meeting that is supposed to go for half an hour; it lasts three hours and ends up taking place over dinner.

Now Katrina and I want to build a life together. It would be nice to have one or two kids. Because of my age, I'm not as focused on this path as Katrina. Somewhere, tucked away at the back of my mind, is the idea that I might be too old. I certainly want a family of my own, but I would probably be okay if it didn't work out that way.

After a year of trying to conceive, we start wondering whether something is wrong. Is there a reason we can't have children? Eventually we get an appointment with a top fertility specialist.

'I'm going to get you pregnant!' this man declares, a little too confidently, when we first find ourselves seated opposite him.

My sperm is tested, no problems there. Katrina has a few basic tests and they can't see anything wrong with her either. At this stage it's almost a novelty for us. We're curious, and content to go along with it all.

Two rounds of intrauterine insemination (IUI) later, and Katrina still isn't pregnant.

All we want to do is conceive a baby. This should be as easy as falling off a log. Instead, this is costing money and taking up a lot of time. The novelty has worn off.

Tense times

Now we are embarking on in vitro fertilisation, and I've discovered that going to these fertility clinics to do your duty is not a pleasant experience. Sometimes I can't help thinking: *This is not what I bargained for.*

'Why don't we adopt?' I ask Katrina.

I was adopted myself; I know I can love an adopted child. Genes aren't important to me.

'I'm not sure about adoption,' Katrina tells me.

'You've got to take me into consideration here too,' I tell her. 'This is just a pain in the arse, going through these medical procedures.'

'I'm willing to look into adoption, but I want to try these other options first,' she says.

So I leave it at that.

Going through the medical procedures is bad enough, but it's so much worse because Katrina is telling other people what we're doing. She explains a lot of the details to her mother, in particular. We're trying to create our own family here, and I'm annoyed that Katrina is so entwined in the family she grew up in. I want some autonomy and space for us. I don't like the feeling that our situation has become public property.

The IVF begins, but we don't even get as far as the implantation stage. Katrina's eggs aren't strong enough. We're told that all the drugs in the world aren't going to change that. We need to look outside our marriage to conceive; we need an egg donor. Katrina's self-esteem takes a big *thwack.*

'I feel as though I'm not a whole person,' she tells me.

We're both shocked, and it takes a bit of time for us to get our heads around the news. But in the end we decide to give egg donation a try. I'm daunted by what is involved, and stressed by our statistically low chance of a successful outcome. But the concept of using someone else's eggs doesn't trouble me. Like I said, genes aren't that important to me.

I've been a bit blasé until this point, but now that we have to involve other people, this all feels like a big deal. I have to commit to this fully. We're on a mission.

Funnily enough, I've been talking to other fathers lately, men who had children in their fifties and sixties. Until now I've had my doubts about becoming a father in my fifties. But everyone I've spoken to says I should just do it. 'It's the best thing in the world,' they tell me. Maybe they're right. Maybe I'll never be truly fulfilled until I become a father.

Irons in the fire

Suddenly Katrina and I feel desperate. We're prepared to pursue any avenue that might bring a child into our family. We're looking for an egg donor, and Katrina is now willing to start the adoption process. She is putting together a scrapbook of our family photos for the adoption agency. There's a shot of us on a beach in Asia. There's a picture of our house. Photos of Katrina's family. We hope the book will show potential birth mothers that our child will have a good life and be exposed to lots of wonderful experiences.

> Maybe they're right. Maybe I'll never be truly fulfilled until I become a father.

We have to provide a family history and our fingerprints to the adoption agency. We undergo a police check and a counsellor visits our house to see if it will be suitable for children. We also register on a waiting list at an IVF clinic for anonymous egg donors. More forms to fill out and doctors and counsellors to speak to. I'm conscious of the fact that we're trying to have a baby. This should be a private thing between two people, but we have agencies and medical experts and all sorts of people getting involved.

The timelines for adoption and egg donation are so long and drawn out. It feels like we're stuck somewhere between the land of newlyweds and the land of parenthood. It's a nowhere kind of place. Limbo.

Egg donation

It could be a long time before we reach the top of the egg donor list.

I'm not hung up on the gene thing, but it would be nice to have a donor from the same gene pool as Katrina, and for our child to experience a relationship with the person who provides this huge gift to us.

I get home from work one night and Katrina says to me, 'I have great news for you.'

'What is it?'

'My cousin has offered to donate her eggs to us!'

'That's fabulous,' I say.

Joanna, who lives on another continent, made the offer without even being asked. If truth be told, if we could have picked anyone in the world to be the donor, it would have been her.

It's Katrina's birthday soon and she's having a big party. We decide to fly Joanna over for the occasion, and attempt an implantation at the same time.

Katrina is juggling a million things at the same time, organising her party, entertaining visitors from out of town, and somehow fitting in her day in hospital. A few people know what we're doing, including my mother-in-law. Everyone has their fingers crossed. I don't like the feeling that we're being watched.

Joanna's procedure is much more involved than anything Katrina or I need to go through. She's such a good soul. She's uncomfortable for a couple of days, but she's in good spirits through the entire process.

During the fortnight following the implantation, Katrina keeps asking me, 'Do you think it has worked?'

I tell her my honest answer: 'I really don't know, but I hope so'.

I'm away on a business trip when Katrina calls me with the results. Even before she says the words, I can tell by her voice that it hasn't worked. Within a couple of days I'm back home, holding her in my arms and sharing her sadness.

We were disappointed when our IUI and IVF attempts failed. But it always felt like we had other options. This time, the news really upsets us. We assume that we can't involve Joanna again; it would be too much to expect someone to go through this process twice.

We go into some serious action. We ramp up our adoption efforts, investigating other adoption agencies we might be able to use. We also start researching other IVF clinics with donor programs. We're still wrestling with the idea of using an anonymous donor. We're not sure how we feel about our child missing out on the chance to know the donor.

> Katrina is very private about her therapy, but I start noticing some changes in her demeanour.

Let's try therapy

My wife reads about a psychotherapist who helps people work through issues from their childhood that might be impeding their ability to conceive.

I know there is a connection between the mind and the body, because whenever I'm stressed I have a bad back that plays up. I'm not sure of the extent of the connection between emotional issues and fertility, but I'm happy for Katrina to try anything that might help. And I'm a big advocate of therapy in general, since I got to know myself a lot better a few years ago when I saw a therapist.

Katrina is very private about her therapy, but I start noticing some changes in her demeanour. She is more sure of herself, and she has a much more positive outlook.

She's in this new headspace when she gets a call from the adoption agency. A girl who is a few months' pregnant wants to give her baby up for adoption. Katrina agrees to talk with her.

When I get home from work that night she has a lot to report.

'The girl is very nice,' she tells me. 'She's understandably confused, but she's sure that she wants to give the baby up.'

Wow! This is real. There is an actual child growing in an actual womb at this moment and it could be ours.

Adoption isn't our first choice. We would prefer to go down the egg donation route, but we're not sure whether we'll have another opportunity to pursue that. So we're excited about this adoption, and we start seeing a counsellor at the agency.

A few weeks later, the birth mother has some medical expenses. We are happy to pay them for her. Then she wants to move out of her parents' home so that she can be in a better psychological space. She asks if we can guarantee her lease and pay her rent. At first we agree to it, but something doesn't smell right. The counsellor tells us that these sorts of requests are common. But I decide to back off, and Katrina agrees. I can see how much the therapy has improved her confidence. A few months ago, I'm not sure she could have walked away from this option with so much certainty.

At least now we have hope. After going through this process we feel confident that we will be able to adopt a child in the future if or when it feels right.

Implanting overseas

Unbelievably, Joanna offers to undergo another egg collection if we're interested.

'You are an absolute saint,' we both tell her over the phone, with huge smiles on our faces. This was not at all expected.

We certainly couldn't ask Joanna to put herself through this again, so we decide this is our last shot. If it doesn't work we're going to call it quits on all the medical procedures and adopt. That gives us an added sense of pressure, but it doesn't feel like a 'bad' kind of pressure. It's more like a strong feeling that more than ever before we really need it to work this time.

Our doctor suggests that it would be best to fly over to be with Joanna, so that she won't be undergoing procedures after a long flight. Great! We get a holiday and an implantation all at once.

Katrina gives me the biggest sign of all that the therapy is changing the way she operates. She decides she's not going to tell anyone this time. She's going to be her own person. We fly out to be with Joanna, and everyone thinks we're just going for a holiday.

I'm excited. Katrina and I are a real team on this – I love that no-one else knows what's going on. But Katrina feels guilty that she hasn't told her mother.

'What will I say if Mum calls or emails while we're away?'

'At any point, if you feel you need to tell her, just tell her,' I say.

But we both agree that this feels a lot easier without the added pressure of family members checking in on us throughout the process.

We have a happy reunion with Joanna and her family. We check out the zoo and take a boat ride around the harbour. While Joanna is having the procedures done, we look after her children for her, taking them to parks and eating ice creams together.

Katrina and I know that we're here for one reason – to have a baby. It feels good to prioritise the procedures, rather than squeezing them in around our busy lives. My work is not interfering. Our social lives aren't interfering.

The first part of the process goes well. To our delight, we end up with three embryos. We can freeze two of them to use at a later date.

The night before the implantation procedure, Katrina and I go to a waterfront restaurant together, just the two of us. With our bellies full, we walk along the docks holding hands, feeling hopeful and nervous, and very close to each other.

Joanna and I are both in the room with Katrina when the procedure takes place. Joanna is on one side, holding Katrina's hand, and I'm on the other side, holding her other hand. We all look up at the screen as they show us via a remote camera the embryo being extracted from a dish with our names on it.

I'm in awe. That might be our baby I'm staring at on the screen.

A few days later we have an emotional farewell with Joanna and we board our return flight. Sitting on the plane, we're all giggly. One of the air hostesses has come across a bunch of wigs, and every time she walks past she has a new one on.

I keep thinking to myself: *Let's hope this works. Let's hope this works.*

Back home, Katrina has a blood test to see whether the embryo has taken.

When she rings up for the results, the lady from the clinic starts reciting a heap of numbers at her: 'Your such-and-such levels are X, and your such-and-such is Y'.

'I just want to know if I'm pregnant or not ...' Katrina says.

'Yeah, you are.'

'Really?'

I see her whole face light up. We both start jumping around and shouting, 'Yea!'

We decide not to tell anyone for the first three months. We feel very protective of this new life, because we've fought so hard and long for it. The only exception is Katrina's family, including Joanna, of course.

When Katrina's mum finds out about the pregnancy, she feels hurt. Excluded.

At first Katrina feels terrible, but she decides to let the issue go. She doesn't want to spend too much time stressing about the past if there is a chance the baby might be affected by those emotions.

Apart from that hiccup, Katrina is so happy being pregnant. She's acting all 'nesty' and nothing in the world worries her. I am devouring books on child rearing, and as the birth draws closer, I'm very content to be the guy who runs errands and does whatever needs to be done.

We organise for Joanna to fly in around the time of the birth.

We really want a natural birth, but due to complications the doctor recommends that we have a caesarean. As I sit holding Katrina's hand, the doctor works away behind a little screen. All of a sudden they hold up this little munchkin. She starts crying – my God, it's the best sound in the world.

I stand side by side with the nurse as she weighs this tiny baby girl. I'm staring at my daughter in a trance, stroking her arm, and she grabs onto my finger with her little hand. It's the sweetest thing in the world.

Joanna comes in to visit us and give her blessing to this new baby. We tell her that we would like her to be our daughter's godmother. And we plan to tell our baby girl right from the start just how special this godmother is. 'Joanna gave a little piece of herself so that we could make you,' we will say.

> Our marriage is completely different ... Before I know it, I am thinking *Why aren't I getting any attention?*

I walk home from the hospital with Joanna, and she lets out a huge sigh. 'It's not my child,' she realises.

We couldn't know until this moment what it would be like for all of us, but there is no question that this baby girl is Katrina's daughter. She's breastfeeding and bonding with her as though that was the way it was always meant to be. Nature has an amazing way of creating that perfect bond between mother and child even though it wasn't biologically perfect to start with. It's a big relief for all of us.

Being a dad

I never knew how all-encompassing it would be to have a child. It's a 24-hour-a-day job.

Our marriage is completely different. We're not going out to dinner any more or doing any of the things we used to do together. Before I know it, I'm thinking, *Why aren't I getting any attention?*

'You've changed,' I tell Katrina. I'm angry with her. Yelling at her. 'You don't give me any of your time. I have to work, and then when I get home I constantly have to do stuff around the house.'

She fires back: 'What about me? I don't get any time for myself, either.'

We're not listening to each other.

I decide to have some sessions with Katrina's psychotherapist. She takes me back to my childhood to help me understand why I'm having these issues as a parent.

I was an only child. My father was my best friend in the world. I remember him taking me to the playground, and I remember riding around on his shoulders feeling so safe and reassured. He died when I was seven. My mother thought she was doing the right thing in keeping me away from his funeral, but it just prolonged the hurt and the emptiness I felt when he left my world.

Mum pretended that everything was okay. But it wasn't. She was consumed by grief and struggled to survive without a man in her life. I was told to be a good boy. I behaved and played quietly so that I wouldn't add to my mother's emotional burdens. But I was a child, and I wasn't getting the love I needed.

Now, here I am a 52-year-old man, and I'm still wanting to be noticed and scooped up and loved by the woman in my life.

For a while we've been thinking about flying back to Joanna's home country to implant the frozen embryos. Maybe my therapy will help our chances, especially if Katrina and I can start to get along better.

Another child?

Katrina tells her family everything about our upcoming procedures, and I'm feeling very sorry for myself. It feels like she's treating them as her family, instead of me.

I can just imagine the news spreading around the family. 'Oh they're trying that again!' Several family members call in regularly wanting to be updated. Katrina feels a lot of pressure to perform. She doesn't want to let all of these people down.

We make the intercontinental trip, but you wouldn't say we are getting along.

Then, at our destination we're told that the quality of the defrosted embryos isn't great. There is only one that is good enough to implant, but even that one isn't looking crash hot. I don't think this is going to work.

Katrina and I are arguing.

I keep saying, 'We should be taking it easy like last time'. But everyone in Joanna's extended family knows we're here, and this trip feels a lot more social.

The relatives say things like: 'You're lucky to have your daughter. Maybe you shouldn't wish so hard for a second child, that way you won't be disappointed if it doesn't happen.'

The doctors need some extra time to get Katrina's hormone levels up. I have to head back home for work, and I feel horrible that I won't be there for the implantation. But I'm not feeling all that supportive, to be honest. My mood has been flat because of all the family involvement and the poor quality of the embryo.

One of Katrina's cousins offers to fly back with her.

'Why would you offer to do that?' I ask her.

'Because we're family. That's what we do.'

Quite involuntarily, tears come to my eyes. I don't know what it means to have a big family. To look out for each other. To belong and to feel loved. I'm envious.

Joanna accompanies Katrina to the implantation procedure. I'm travelling around for my work, and my communication with Katrina is sparse.

With Katrina back home, we find out that the embryo didn't take. We're disappointed, but we're not entirely surprised.

More than anything else, I'm upset that Katrina's getting all the attention, and I'm still being forgotten.

Dynamic shift

I continue with my therapy, and Katrina and I also do a number of sessions as a couple. We explore the issues that are underlying our arguments, bad moods and criticisms of each other. Before too long we can see that these things all stem from neediness on both sides. We can see that it will work much better if we start supporting each other rather than cutting each other down.

I realise that most of my issues with Katrina come down to one thing. I'm so sad that she has her parents and I don't. My mum passed away when I was a teenager. I've been alone in the world for a long time.

Now that I can see the cause of my angst towards Katrina's family, I suddenly see them for who they really are. I no longer feel threatened by them.

We've been living a long distance from Katrina's family for the past few years, and she is not happy about this. I decide we should move back to be closer to them. I don't mind a long commute if it means that she'll be more content.

The kindness of strangers

Just as we start to consider our options for finding another egg donor, we receive a serendipitous phone call. It has been three years since we put our names down on that waiting list for an egg donor. We had almost forgotten that we'd done it.

'You're at the top of the list,' they tell us.

We only have a few days to decide whether to take up the offer. We grapple with the anonymity issue, but we're comforted by the fact that our child would be able to meet the donor when he or she turns eighteen, according to local laws.

We're given some information about our potential donor. She has blonde hair and is a nurse. The fact that she is in a caring role is really important to us. We have a really good feeling about it.

We decide to repeat the thing that worked so well for us the first time around – we keep this whole thing a secret.

On the day I'm required to provide the sperm, I can't help noticing a blonde lady in the waiting room. I wonder if it's her.

A few days later Katrina goes in to have two embryos implanted. The embryologist tells us that they are the strongest she has ever seen. The walls are thick and on a scale of one to ten, one of them is a ten. The other is a nine.

Katrina and I are full of confidence. Somehow we feel this is meant to be.

She asks me, 'Do you think it will work?'

'I'm sure of it,' I tell her. And I mean it.

I'm sitting at work a couple of weeks later when Katrina calls me.

'It worked,' she tells me.

'I told you it would!'

By law, we're not allowed to provide any sort of letter or gift to the donor. We ask the counsellor at the clinic to send this lady some flowers on our behalf. That's the only way we can convey to this woman our immense gratitude.

Today

I'm now a father of two daughters. I absolutely love having a family of my own. After being without that for so long, it means everything to me. When I walk through the door after a day at work, my older daughter runs up to me and I put her up on my shoulders. I only recently remembered that my dad used to do the same thing with me.

> A few days later Katrina goes in to have two embryos implanted. The embryologist tells us that they are the strongest she has ever seen.

I'm still not used to living with so much noise, and I miss having time to myself. But I'm continuing to see our psychotherapist, and she's helping me be a better husband and father all the time. I only wish I'd started to see her before we had our first baby, I would have been much better prepared for parenthood.

When we were trying to conceive, I often had a macho voice in my head telling me this wasn't really my problem. It wasn't my plumbing, so to speak.

My big lesson in all of this is that a family is made by two people. If you want to be a father who is involved in family life, it all starts at the conception.

It was fundamental for me to realise that my desperation to be loved when I was a child ended up playing out in my relationship with Katrina. She wasn't able to become pregnant – either time – until I stopped being focused on my own needs and instead gave her all of my love, support and commitment.

* Real names were replaced with pseudonyms in this story.

Editor's notes

Page vii: '... recent studies ... have shown improved pregnancy outcomes in women participating in stress reduction programs': For example, Domar, A, Seibel, M and Benson, H, 'The mind/body program for infertility: a new behavioral treatment approach for women with infertility', *Fertility and Sterility*, vol. 53, no. 2, 1990, pp: 246–9. Also: Berga, S, Marcus, M, Loucks, T, Hlastala, S, Ringham, R and Krohn, M, 'Recovery of ovarian activity in women with functional hypothalamic amenorrhea who were treated with cognitive behavior therapy', *Fertility and Sterility*, vol. 80, no. 4, 2003, p: 976.

Page viii: '... subjective emotional distress can impact on conception even in the absence of measurable changes in stress hormones': Sanders, K and Bruce, N, 'A prospective study of psychosocial stress and fertility in women', *Human Reproduction*, vol. 12, 1997, pp: 2324–9.

Page 1: '... the level of stress experienced by infertility patients is often similar to the stress endured by people suffering from serious illnesses such as cancer': Domar, A, Zuttermeister, P and Friedman, R., 'The psychological impact of infertility: a comparison with patients with other medical conditions', *Journal of Psychosomatic Obstetrics and Gynaecology*, vol. 14, Suppl., 1993, pp: 45–52.

Page 13: 'I also read a beautiful book ...': Diamant, Anita, *The Red Tent*, Allen & Unwin, St Leonards, NSW, 1998.

Page 16: 'The pressure is getting to Dave, and sometimes he can't perform': 'Fertility problem stress' increases marital conflict and decreases sexual self-esteem and satisfaction with one's own sexual performance: Andrews, F, Abbey, A and Halman, J, 'Stress from infertility, marriage factors, and subjective well-being of wives and husbands', *Journal of Health and Social Behavior*, vol. 32, no. 3, 1991, pp: 238–53.

Page 36: '**... I told him how much happier I was**': A study of women who had experienced at least one unsuccessful IVF cycle showed that those who were not depressed before starting IVF treatment had a conception rate twice as high as women who were depressed before treatment: Thiering, P, Beaurepaire, J, Jones, M, Saunders, D and Tennant, C, 'Mood state as a predictor of treatment outcome after in vitro fertilization/ embryo transfer technology (IVF/ET)', *Journal of Psychosomatic Research*, vol. 37, 1993, pp: 481–91.

Page 62: '**Keith thinks my obsession is dangerously affecting my physical and emotional wellbeing**': A prolonged condition of stress may be associated with high amounts of activated T-cells in the peripheral blood, and this may be associated with reduced implantation rates for women undergoing IVF embryo transfers: Gallinelli, A, Roncaglia, R, Matteo, ML, Ciaccio, I, Volpe, A and Facchinetti, F, 'Immunological changes and stress are associated with different implantation rates in patients undergoing in vitro fertilization – embryo transfer', *Fertility and Sterility*, vol. 76, no. 1, 2001, pp: 85–91.

Page 112: '**The only time I relaxed was in my sleep**': According to research conducted in South Africa, there is potentially a correlation between sufferers of endometriosis and a personality type involving 'time urgent perfectionism': Rodrigues, A, Wolff, E and Wolff, M, *Faster, Better, Sicker – Time Urgency Perfectionism Stress*, Xtime, South Africa, 2004.

Page 121: '**His support during that final round of IVF helped me drop a lot of the anxiety I'd had in previous rounds**': In a study of 818 Danish couples, women who reported greater levels of marital distress required more assisted reproduction cycles to conceive (a median of three) than women reporting less marital distress (a median of two): Boivin, J and Schmidt, L, 'Infertility-related stress in men and women predicts treatment outcome one year later', *Fertility and Sterility*, vol. 83, no. 6, 2005, pp: 1745–52.

Page 125: '**Looking back, we probably didn't discuss it fully**': Difficulties in partner communication lead to high 'fertility problem stress' for both men and women: Schmidt, L, Holstein, B, Christensen, U and Boivin, J, 'Communication and coping as predictors of fertility problem stress: cohort study of 816 participants who did not achieve a delivery after 12 months of fertility treatment', *Human Reproduction*, vol. 20, 2005, pp: 3248–56.

Page 139: '**In the end, a book called *Miscarriage* ... saved me**': Regan, Lesley, *Miscarriage: What Every Woman Needs to Know – A Positive New Approach*, Bloomsbury, London, 1997.

Page 180: '**Just after Mum died, I found a book ... called *The Whole Person Fertility Program***': Payne, Niravi, *The Whole Person Fertility Program*, Three Rivers Press, New York, 1997.

Bibliography

Domar, A, 'Infertility and the mind/body connection', *The Female Patient*, Signature Series, 2005.

Domar, A, Clapp, D, Slawsby, E, Dusek, J, Kessel, B and Freizinger, M, 'The impact of group psychological interventions on pregnancy rates in infertile women', *Fertility and Sterility*, vol. 73, no. 4, 2000, pp: 805–11.

Domar, A, Zuttermeister, P and Friedman, R, 'Distress and conception in infertile women: a complementary approach', *Journal of the American Medical Women's Association*, vol. 54, no. 4, 1999, pp: 196–9.

Eastburn, Lynsi, *It's Conceivable! Hypnosis for Fertility*, Trafford Publishing, Victoria, Canada, 2006.

Ford, Judy, *It Takes Two: Reproducing Naturally Today*, Environmental and Genetic Solutions, Adelaide, Australia, 1997.

Lapane, K, Zierler, S, Lasater, T, Stein, M, Barbour, M and Hume, A, 'Is a history of depressive symptoms associated with an increased risk of infertility in women?', *Psychosomatic Medicine*, vol. 57, no. 6, 1995, pp: 509–13.

Payne, Naravi, *The Whole Person Fertility Program: A Revolutionary Mind–Body Process to Help You Conceive*, Three Rivers Press, New York, 1997.

Pert, Candace, *Molecules of Emotion: The Science Behind Mind–Body Medicine*, Scribner, New York, 1997.

Sharkey, Ruth, *Fertile Fathers*, Ruth Sharkey, Queensland, Australia, 2002.

Sharkey, Ruth, *Ruth Sharkey's Guide to Natural Conception*, Ruth Sharkey, Tasmania, Australia, 2004.

Acknowledgements

When you have a vision of something you want to create, it's amazing how many people offer the encouragement, contacts and resources you need to make it happen.

The first person to offer encouragement for this project was my husband, Ted. You believed in me always, Teddy! Thank you for sharing every aspect of this journey with me.

Thanks to my family (Keoghs, Quins and Ryans) for your excitement about this project. Thank you, Mum, for your editing, for nurturing my inner-writer always, and for being thrilled to bits every time I told you about this book. And to Dad for being willing to do absolutely whatever you could to help me.

Thank you to my gorgeous friends for really getting behind me. Thanks especially to everyone who brought potential stories or fertility experts to my attention. And thank you to those friends and family members who reviewed chapters for me (especially Leeza, Lisa, Varsha and Eynas).

Thanks to Gin, Nat, Nicole, Heidi and Pip for babysitting Declan.

How can I properly express my gratitude to the women and men who shared their stories in this book? I feel a huge amount of love for each of you. Such a privilege to be trusted with the most intimate details of your struggles and joys. It has been incredibly humbling to receive your support for this book. So thank you all – and thank you to your partners. I hope that you can share in the fulfilment I've experienced by writing these words. Let's hope they find their way to those who need them.

A special acknowledgement to Costa Zouliou, who chose to write his own story. I can claim credit only for the editing of that entertaining piece of prose.

A huge thank you to all of the fertility and health practitioners who spoke with me about their work. They include: obstetrician/gynaecologist Dr Ian Mayes; international leader in mind–body medicine Dr Alice Domar; natural fertility advisor Kerry Hampton; hypnotherapist and clinical psychologist Elizabeth Muir; psychotherapist Niravi Payne; healer Mary Malady; journey practitioner Yollana Shore; naturopath and medical herbalist Francesca Naish; baby yoga instructor Suzanne Swan; naturopath Doreen Schwegler; naturopath Melissa MacDonald and her partner Michael Bonett; psychologist Gayle Crespy; art therapist Veronica Hughes; herbalist Ruth Sharkey and geneticist Dr Judy Ford.

Thank you, Rex Finch, for running with this idea. I'm extremely grateful to you for taking on the business side of this project and helping me to make this dream come true.

Thanks to my editor, Samantha! You've been incredibly ace to work with. A huge support.

Finally, thank you to everyone at Human Potentials, especially Emma Tyree, for everything you've helped me to learn. Because of my work with you guys, I was able to take this book to a whole new level, and foster some magical relationships along the way.

Index

Also available from Vermilion

The Optimum Fertility Diet
by Dr Caroline Shreeve

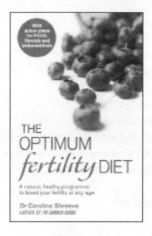

The complete dietary and lifestyle advice included in this practical guide will help couples with no fertility issues who want to plan for a family; support infertile couples who are losing hope of ever having a baby naturally; and inspire single women in their 30s and 40s who want to preserve their peak fertility until Mr Right shows up.

With chapters on vitamins and supplements; fertility super foods; enhancing the fertility of men and older women; and relaxation and exercise, this comprehensive guide is for all couples who want to conceive naturally. Dr Caroline Shreeve also includes menu plans, delicious recipes and a 'Fertility Action Plan' for women with conditions such as PCOS, fibroids and endometriosis.

Accessible, sensitive and straightforward, *The Optimum Fertility Diet* will boost your chances of conceiving the old-fashioned way.

£10.99　　　　　　　ISBN 9780091924010　　　　　　　www.rbooks.co.uk

Planning A Baby?
by Dr Sarah Brewer

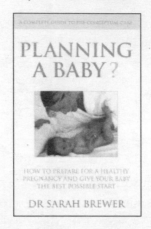

Research has shown that good nutrition and wellbeing during the first few weeks of gestation – often before the mother is even aware she is pregnant – can affect the baby a long way into the future. *Planning A Baby?* is all about giving your baby the best possible start in life, teaching you how to take maximum care of your health in the six important months before your new child is even conceived, to optimise the chances of having a healthy baby.

In this completely updated and revised edition, Dr Sarah Brewer provides the latest groundbreaking research and gives advice on contraceptive advances, lifestyle factors that affect early pregnancy, the necessary vitamins and minerals needed for optimal development, advice for vegetarians, sperm health and much much more.

Planning A Baby? aims to give potential parents all the tools they require before embarking on one of life's greatest adventures – conception, pregnancy and the birth of a healthy baby.

£8.99   ISBN 9780091898489   www.rbooks.co.uk